LIFE, DEATH,
AND
THE DOCTOR

LIFE, DEATH,
AND
THE DOCTOR

Louis Lasagna, M.D.

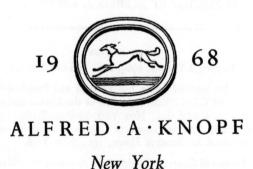

19 68

ALFRED · A · KNOPF
New York

To my mother and father

FOREWORD

THIS BOOK deals with health problems of critical importance to both the medical profession and society. The
problems are neither new nor secret. Why, then, a book about
them? I have undertaken the task because first of all these
difficulties deserve continuing debate and reappraisal, in the
hope that society may find the solutions that escape us at present. A further justification is the conviction that there is some
merit in a book intended for the public but written by a physician. The doctor is both a member of his profession and a
member of society. This leads to important ambivalences, but
it also provides a unique opportunity to attack problems facing
physicians and laymen alike.

This is not an "anti-doctor" book. There have been enough
of those written of late to last us for the next decade. Given
the opportunity to choose a career again, I would still aim for a
life of patient care, education, and research. I find being a
doctor exciting and rewarding, and I admire many of my colleagues as scientists and people. But because of my respect and
affection, I find the apathy, ignorance, or obstructionism of the
profession on certain important issues all the more distressing.
One of my hopes is that airing these issues will improve the
quality of the debate. Doctors tend to talk to doctors about
medical issues, and laymen to laymen. The result is misunder-
standing, a lack of appreciation of the other's point of view,

and failure to pool forces against the common enemies of disease and death.

The plan of the book is a simple one, even if the topics are extraordinarily complex. Since the doctor is a key figure throughout, the book begins with a description of the background of the physician and tries to point out both how he is uniquely fitted to serve society and why he is not serving it as well as he might.

The next three chapters in Section I deal with "educational" problems. These first discuss the need for revising and updating medical-school training, then the problem of maintaining the doctor's knowledge and skills after school and hospital training, and finally the educational and corrective measures required to prevent disability and death from such environmental hazards as noise, vehicular accidents, air pollution, ionizing radiation, and cigarette smoking.

Section II discusses some fundamental aspects of life and death, including the population explosion, world food needs, birth control, abortion, sterilization, severe mental retardation, senescence, and euthanasia.

Section III concerns interactions between medicine and the law, including the patient-doctor contract, the Good Samaritan controversy, informed consent, professional secrecy, court testimony, and legal restraints on patients afflicted with insanity. The last chapter analyzes the morass of moral, penal, and medical issues involved in drug abuse.

It would be both surprising and depressing if readers were to find nothing to disagree with in my book. Since the issues discussed are as dynamic as they are important, controversy and uncertainty are more appropriate than rigid attitudes. My own opinions about these matters are constantly changing, sometimes radically. While I hope to educate the reader, I also hope that his response to the book will contribute as much to my education.

September 1967   LOUIS LASAGNA

ACKNOWLEDGMENTS

SOME OF THE MATERIAL in this book has been published previously in the following periodicals: *The New Republic* ("Why Are Doctors Out of Step?"), the *Journal of Chronic Diseases* ("The Investigator's Responsibility to the Patient," "A Matter of Perspective," and "Is Narcotic Addiction a Chronic Disease?"), the *Yale Journal of Biology and Medicine* ("The Mind and Morality of the Doctor"), *Clinical Research* ("Cricket, Critics, Conformity, and Curmudgeonship"), *The New York Times Magazine* ("The Control of Heredity: Dream or Nightmare?," "Fearfully and Wonderfully Made," and "The G.P. Is Still Needed"), *Fact* ("The Misleading Advertisements of Bayer Aspirin"), and *The Catholic Digest* ("Are We Poisoning Our World?").

I am indebted to many people for many things, although I do not wish to imply that any errors in this book should be blamed on them. To begin with, I am grateful to medical students at a number of universities in this country and abroad for the opportunity to discuss matters of interest to society and to the profession with them; they have provided both education and inspiration. I am indebted to Jeanne Ridley and Mindel Sheps for the opportunity to participate in the University of Pittsburgh Symposium on "Public Health and Population Change," which gave me my first real insight into the complexities of the population-control problem. (The contents of that symposium have been published by the University of Pittsburgh Press and are well worth reading.) I wish to thank the individuals responsible for the Kaiser Foundation Symposium on "Man Against Himself," where I had the chance to meet with, listen to, and learn from such people as Rachel Carson, Peter Medawar, Harrison Brown, and E. Cuyler Hammond.

A number of other meetings, including the White House conferences on drug abuse and health and the Massachusetts Institute of Technology summer conference on medical education, have helped to familiarize me with some of the topics discussed.

I am grateful to friends, colleagues, and experts such as Robert Hall, Harold Rosen, and André Hellegers, for their discussions of the problems of abortion; Christopher Tietze, whose erudite writings have illuminated the field of contraception techniques; Reubin Andres, who so kindly read and criticized the section on aging; and the late, remarkable Mason Lord and my teacher and friend David Seegal for providing perspective on the problems of the elder citizen and the patient with chronic disease.

A cherished friend and able lawyer, Alfred Bressler, helped greatly with his comments on the sections dealing with the law. These sections also owe much to the comprehensive book *The Law and Medical Practice*, by Burke Shartel and Marcus L. Plant, and to the writings of Yale Katz, Manfred Guttmacher, and Samuel Bessman.

For the section on drug abuse I am heavily indebted to the work of such people as Harris Isbell, Abraham Wikler, Nathan Eddy, Henry K. Beecher, J. M. von Felsinger, Alfred Lindesmith, Isidor Chein, and Jack Mendelson.

James Coleman and Harold Wilensky provided some imaginative insights into the relationship between the medical profession and the public. I am grateful for many things to Houston Peterson, including his assignment, to an admiring

Rutgers senior in 1943, of the work of John Dewey referred to in the Epilogue.

It would be impossible to express my indebtedness to the hundreds of medical journals, newspapers, and books consulted over the last two decades in preparation for this book, but I would like to pay special tribute to *Medical Tribune* and *Medical World News,* the *Journal of Medical Education,* Norman E. Hines's *Medical History of Contraception,* and Bernard Strehler's informative *Time, Cells, and Aging.*

Finally, special thanks are extended to Dorothy Burns, Ruth Kimmerer, and Susan Wills for their patience and ability in preparing the manuscript.

CONTENTS

Part I

THE DOCTOR, HIS TRAINING, AND THE CHALLENGE OF NEW RESPONSIBILITIES

I

Is the Doctor Fit
to Serve Society?

I N 1965 Dr. Ivan L. Bennett, Jr., Professor of Pathology at
Johns Hopkins University, gave the convocation address
to the graduating class of Hopkins medical students. Its title,
"Strangers and Brothers," was taken from the C. P. Snow
novel, and was used to signify that whereas the members of the
medical profession are in a sense brothers, the inclination of
many doctors to obstruct social change tends to make them
strangers to the public and to colleagues with a greater social
conscience. The speech was hard-hitting and abundantly laced
with damning quotes from leaders of local and national medical associations. Bennett warned: "We must recognize that
medicine is not now and never has been our private preserve
but is something in which all people have a vital stake."

At the reception after the convocation, there was a certain
coolness evident on the part of the physician-fathers present,
but the temperature warmed up considerably when irate doctors in the community began writing letters to the Baltimore
Sun, protesting the "attack." Even laymen entered the fray,
defending their doctors, both live and dead. By midsummer

Professor Bennett remarked, on his way back to Baltimore from a conference in Boston, "I hope another kindly old general practitioner hasn't died since I've been gone."

There seems little question that the Bennetts are in the minority in the medical profession, but there is more than a little restlessness among physicians about their role in society. A few years ago I wrote an article entitled "Why Are Doctors Out of Step?" for *The New Republic.* It evoked a mail response modest in quantity but passionate in tone. From California came the following: "The frustration you express is shared by several of my close friends who are young physicians of liberal bent who dare not express their sentiments . . . for fear of economic reprisal."

A Texas doctor wrote: "I wonder if most doctors are not ignorant of their social responsibilities. . . . There was no instruction in, and little discussion of, the ethical problems of patient care during medical school. Any consideration of a social ethic for doctors was out of the question."

A physician in Iowa was prompted to say: "Even though we all mill around in the same cultural milieu, I somehow expect physicians to be proponents of a more meaningful society, for theirs is a unique position of influence which can engender action on ideals. To see such Gulliverian strength bound down by rigidity, inflexibility, medical political strategy, [and] personal power is maddening."

Talking with students at such diverse places as the University of Pennsylvania, Stanford, Johns Hopkins, the University of Southern California, Wisconsin, Minnesota, Harvard, and Yale, I have repeatedly been struck by the "welcome ration of disquietude" in their ranks. Many are disturbed by the feeling that they are not being prepared for responsible scientific and social citizenship.

To understand better the current state of affairs, it may help to examine briefly the origins and training of the modern doctor. While a single stereotype is impossible to construct, certain generalizations can be made with reasonable assurance. Medical students are unquestionably superior, intellectually, to the "average man." They have had to run several academic gauntlets in order to be admitted to professional school—first to get accepted to a good college or university (an obscure or second-rate school will seriously handicap them later), then to graduate from college, and finally to satisfy medical-school admissions committees that among all those competing for the vacant slots, they deserve enrollment.

One out of five medical-school freshmen is married; by the senior year three out of five are. They tend to come from upper-income families. Only 15 per cent of all medical students are from families whose income is less than $5,000, whereas in the general population 36 per cent of all families are in that bracket. And 14 per cent of medical students come from the 1 per cent of families with income in excess of $25,000 a year. Over two fifths of medical students have fathers who are professional men, of whom about one third are physicians. There is a disproportionately high representation of medical students from larger communities.

It costs a lot of money to be a medical student: the average expense in a 1964 survey was $2,713 per year for the single ones, $4,797 for the married without children, and still more for those with children.[1] Most medical students receive substantial financial help from their families; many also derive aid from working wives, scholarships, and loans. One out of seven students comes to medical school owing money for college debts, the average being $1,500. By the time they are seniors, almost half have debts, the average being $3,000. Clearly, this expense poses serious obstacles to would-be doctors from poorer families, just as it helps to explain both the economic conservatism of the average doctor and his keen concern with matters related to his income.

An interesting analysis of medical students at the Uni-

[1] These expenses have risen in many schools since 1964.

versity of Edinburgh has important implications both for the selection of students and for their ultimate role in medicine. The Scottish researchers attempted to see what characteristics clustered together, and they concluded that the students fell into four general categories. The first was the "adequate graduate"—a realist, well adjusted, calm, able to relate to patients but not especially interested in their emotional problems, convinced of the importance of money.

The second, the "limited graduate," does not like working with people, is harshly critical of patients, rejects nonorganic forms of illness, and actually spends considerable energy warding off patients whom he regards as undesirable. A professional family background was common in this group and may explain the choice of medicine as a career. The third type, the "research-oriented graduate," is not in medicine for financial gain or social status, is mature, objective, technically competent, with a well-planned professional future.

The fourth type, the "patient-centered graduate," wants contact with the sick, resents the lack of such contact in his early years, and is filled with a strong urge to understand and to respond to the needs of his patients. Technically not especially proficient, he does have research interests, which are not, however, "experimental" or "basic science" in nature.

If such clusters of traits and interests can in fact be reliably identified, medical schools should presumably tailor the student's training and direction, lest society end up with doctors who are both frustrated and a threat to the well-being of those in their care. Sir George Pickering, Regius Professor of Medicine at Oxford, has observed: "In the many excellent reports on education . . . during the last thirty years . . . I can recall none that deals with the preservation, let alone the enhancement, of the ethos of medicine . . . No one is failed because he is unkind to his patients."

Once out of medical school, the doctor can head for a variety of careers. Of the 300,000 or so physicians in the United

States, perhaps 15,000 are retired or not in practice and some 25,000 are working for the government. Less than two thirds are in private practice, a proportion that has steadily declined over the years. In 1931, for example, 86 per cent of all physicians were private practitioners, and by 1949 it was down to 75 per cent.

About 17 per cent are in hospital service, 5 per cent in teaching, administration, or research, and 2 per cent in laboratory or preventive medicine. During the last thirty years there has been a strong trend toward full-time specialization, group practice, hospital-based service, and federal service.

The average doctor in practice works hard—more than fifty hours a week, most of it in his office, hospital, or clinic, very little on house calls. He spends seven hours a week in recreation, and takes about two weeks off per year for vacation. About two thirds lose no days of work in an entire year, and another 20 per cent lose five days or less. By contrast, the average American male loses a week of work per year.

Doctors incur disease as a result of their work—infections, allergic rashes, exposure to radiation. Although the doctor starts his practice in good health, he thereafter often fails to maintain the standards of medical care he advocates for patients and neglects to have routine physical examinations, urinalyses, blood tests, and chest X rays. Doctors also show the same distressing tendency as laymen to put off seeking treatment, be it for hypertension, peptic ulcer, or cancer. Indeed, there is evidence that delays in diagnosing or treating cancer may be even longer for physicians than for laymen.

Doctors have more coronary disease than dentists or lawyers, but there are large differences from one medical specialty to another. Dermatologists and pathologists, for example, who are perhaps under the least stress, show a prevalence of coronary heart disease less than half that of anesthesiologists and general practitioners.

The doctor also suffers special jeopardy in regard to military service. He is subject—along with other health personnel—to a discriminatory draft. The "doctor draft" was orginally established in 1950 "to insure the Armed Forces an adequate number of physicians, dentists, and allied specialists." At first, doctors up to age fifty were eligible; the upper limit is now thirty-five years, but deferment on the basis of family needs or physical defects is almost unknown. The doctor is "invited" by his Selective Service Board to accept a commission within thirty days, and those who decline can be (and have been) inducted as privates in the Army.

To compensate for the long hours and the arduous road to medical practice, society has rewarded the doctor in several ways. A national sampling of adults by the University of Chicago's National Opinion Research Center showed that physicians enjoy more prestige than any other occupational group in the United States except Supreme Court Justices. The public thus rates doctors above nuclear physicists, state governors, Cabinet members, college professors, U.S. Congressmen, corporation directors, bankers, and creative and performing artists. In a *Newsweek* poll, 74 per cent of Americans expressed "a great deal of confidence" in doctors, the highest rating received by any of the seventeen professional groups listed. (By contrast, only 45 per cent had such confidence in the clergy and 22 per cent in advertising men.)

More tangible is the high income of the doctor. A 1965 Department of Labor study of the nation's male workers showed physicians at the top of the heap, with a median salary of $14,561 per year. This was almost $2,000 more than the figure for business managers and $4,000 more than that for lawyers. Clergymen, who go to school almost as long as doctors do, showed a median salary of $4,000 per year.

In view of the origins and economic history of the medical profession, it is perhaps not surprising that politically, most doctors are conservative. During the 1964 Presidential campaign, in which the country elected Lyndon B. Johnson by a

resounding margin, polls of physicians (except for psychiatrists) showed the overwhelming majority of them planning to
vote for Barry Goldwater.

Not only did most doctors oppose Johnson; some seriously
objected to the fact that anyone dared to endorse him. John T.
Connor, later Secretary of Commerce, was an active Johnson-
ite while president of the drug company Merck Sharp and
Dohme. Two physicians distributed a letter urging all doctors
to boycott Merck products, and one Tennessee doctor announced after the election that he would no longer prescribe
Merck drugs. He told druggists in his area to call him before
refilling any prescriptions for Merck products, so that he could
substitute drugs of other companies. Such actions prompted
Medical Tribune, an independent medical newspaper, to edi-
torialize: "We know of no disease that is strictly Republican
or Democratic, of no symptoms of given political coloration,
and no medical suffering that is the exclusive preserve of any
political party. . . . A pharmaceutical house must be judged on
the merits of its products and not by the politics of its officers
or employees."

In Fort Wayne, Indiana, Senator Birch Bayh canceled a
speech before the local Pharmacists' Association because doctors had warned pharmacists to stay away from the meeting,
lest they suffer harsh economic reprisals. Ironically, Bayh had
planned a nonpolitical speech on the national shortage of
medical and paramedical personnel. The Senator pointedly
remarked that organized medicine had ample opportunity to
make itself heard on issues affecting its self-interest through
"its sixty public relations men, its Washington lobby, its thirteen journals, newspapers and magazines, its Political Action
Committee, and its annual budget of $22,500,000."

A poll of my medical-school class on the fifteenth anni-
versary of our graduation revealed an interesting reaction to
the question "What are the most important medical problems
of today?" Some considered the population explosion, public

health in underdeveloped countries, and cancer to be most important, but the most popular responses centered around the theme of "socialized" medicine, with such suggestions as: "Prevent a welfare state," "Avoid socialized medicine," "Get the government out of medicine."

What are the satisfactions of a medical career for the practicing doctor? A recent survey of two hundred Cleveland physicians indicated that the "greatest satisfaction" was "giving help and care," followed by "professional role," "intellectual thoroughness," "consistency of personal and professional ethics," "professional autonomy," "clean working conditions," "right conduct," "being in charge," and "status in the community."

The most important dissatisfactions related to public criticism of doctors and loss of prestige. Other dissatisfactions, in order of importance, were "refractory patients," "not keeping up," "extraneous demands," "impersonal patients," "not being paid," "restrictions on professional independence," and "troubled conscience."

Most of the items of greatest interest to the doctors concerned the emotional side of the patient-doctor relationship. Much of the doctor's gratification appears to come from relating personally to the patient and being able to help and care for him. The doctor is likely to be frustrated and unhappy when the patient is not a "good" patient—when he is "uncooperative," does not "want" to get well, can't get well because he suffers from a hopeless disease, is ungrateful, or shows lack of confidence. Interestingly, the doctors in the sample rarely saw any dissatisfactions as arising from their *own* limitations. If the patient-doctor relationship breaks down, or never develops, the fact is attributed to forces outside the doctor's control. The doctor is, in his own mind, blameless.

If the doctor seems to be a bundle of contradictions and paradoxes, it is not surprising. He lives in a world sharp with the horns of multiple dilemmas. The problems just described relate to the doctor in practice. But the lot of the physician is still further complicated if he happens also to function as a scientist.

In his training, the doctor is brought into contact with two levels of medical activity—that of the research scientist and that of the healer. The distinction is both troublesome and real. One reads that "medical experimentation takes place continually in every doctor's office," and that "the therapy of disease is an experimental aspect of medicine," but in point of fact, the practice of medicine and the pursuit of a scientific problem are not the same.

The physician is primarily concerned with the patient as a patient; he wants to get the patient well as quickly as possible, with a minimum of discomfort, inconvenience, risk, and cost. In the practice of his art the practitioner has to use any measure he considers justified. He is concerned with what works, not with contributions to the body of scientific data.

For the investigator, the primary emphasis is on research. This does not mean that he need be callous or reckless; patients who are in an experiment are likely to be more carefully observed and cared for than if they were not. (It is, in fact, usually safer to predict that patient care will improve as the result of a carefully designed experiment than that exciting new scientific information will emerge.) Researchers have usually had the advantage of intensive training, experience, and the intellectual discipline of an academic atmosphere. Further, the patient may be better served by the restraint observed in therapeutic approach by the critical experimentalist. Often in controlled trials, for example, the placebo-treated patients turn out to be the lucky ones, as the new "remedy" proves to be toxic as well as ineffective.

Notwithstanding the admirable qualities of many research-oriented physicians, however, there still remains an important difference in orientation between the practicing physician and the physician-investigator. Take, for example, the patient with metastatic cancer. Here is a serious disease for which we lack good treatment. There would seem to be no ethical problem in giving a new compound, which may do some good, to a patient who desperately needs help. Yet the situation is only superficially simple.

Those cancer patients who are the first to receive an investigational drug often fail to obtain significant therapeutic benefit, and early pharmacologic trials are likely to entail a certain amount of serious risk from the powerful poisons generally required to treat malignant disease. In such a situation, therefore, the physician might well say "No" to the earliest trial of a new drug, whereas the investigator might say "Yes."

If one then considers the treatment of pain or insomnia, where we have remedies that, while not perfect, are excellent and safe, what is the physician to say? Statistically, there is no question but that the patient has a better chance of adequate relief if given a standard and accepted drug rather than an untried one, no matter how impressive a case for research can be made from the standpoint of society's long-term needs.

The young doctor is confused early in his training by attempts to reconcile the interests and attitudes of his preclinical teachers with the job he has chosen for life—the care of the sick. Because of their nonclinical backgrounds and interests, these professors tend to ignore or denigrate the world of the clinic and the practicing doctor. They seem bent on reducing everything to "fundamental" chemical and physical cellular processes, unaware of the sterility of this ambition. (As H. J. Muller has so pungently put it: "To say . . . that a man is made up of certain chemical elements is a satisfactory description only for those who intend to use him as fertilizer.") The self-esteem of the doctor in practice is hardly likely to be inflated by his having been in an environment dominated by molecular biologists during his formative medical school years.

The physician is also susceptible to the anxieties posed by trying to serve the individual and society at the same time—a dilemma facing us all but of special significance to the doctor because of the way he can manipulate life and death. In J. Bronowski's words, ". . . the problem of every society is to find a compromise between man and men." Two examples may illustrate the problem.

Since the population explosion is one of the world's major threats, the day is probably not far off when physicians will have to help limit their own families as well as those of their patients. But science has made available chemicals and hormone preparations capable of stimulating the human ovary to release an egg for fertilization. For many women suffering from infertility, these drugs represent the possibility of bearing a child. I cannot conceive of any physician helping to solve the population problem by trying to keep such drugs off the market, or away from his patients.

In 1957 the British Committee on Radiological Hazards studied the doses of radiation received by the population of Great Britain as the result of mass miniature radiography of the chest. This survey was calculated to have added perhaps 20 cases of leukemia to the 2,500 in the "normal" yearly total. On the credit side, many cases of remediable disease were detected, including 18,000 cases of pulmonary tuberculosis. Lord Adrian commented: "The 20 deaths from leukemia were no more than a remote possibility, but if they were a certainty would they have been too high a price to pay for the early detection of tuberculosis in 18,000 people?" In the abstract, perhaps the answer might be "No"; for the person with the leukemia, the answer is "Yes."

The honest physician is expected, by many people, to act with godlike omniscience, although he knows how fallible he often is. His every day is filled with grasping at elusive medical hints and whisperings. Many sick patients do not present simple, straightforward problems. There are often alternative diagnostic possibilities and alternative courses of therapeutic action from which the physician must choose.

The doctor, unless he lacks all sense of history, is cognizant of the passing character of much that he considers to be hard scientific truth. In an address to the Royal Society of Medicine entitled "The Discards of Surgery," Sir Ian Fraser recalled—without nostalgia—the passage of outmoded instruments and procedures:

> It is delightful to see certain instruments of torture disappearing. For years an unpleasant compression instrument called a tongue forceps was always on the anaesthetist's table. To hold a slimy tongue successfully it had to grip so hard that it reduced the latter to a swollen mass of raw flesh. It differed little in shape or indeed in appearance from a similar instrument used at one time at the other end of the body. Piles may be expendable but the tongue is not. The simple rubber airway does this all so much better and with no trauma. . . .
>
> My first consultant appointment was to a children's hospital, and I blush to think what I did to cases of Hirschsprung's disease in those days—a lumbar puncture with spinal anaesthesia. What hope was there of that ever doing any permanent good?
>
> Lumbar sympathectomy on the left side and later on the right side was advocated, and finally we resected the distended portion of gut, leaving the contracted aganglionic segment behind. This was surgery at its worst.

In view of the uncertainties constantly facing him, it is imperative for the doctor to develop a sense of critique, but the average physician is limited in his ability to examine conflicting data critically. In an interesting book that appeared in 1966, *Controversies in Internal Medicine*, experts took violently contrasting stands on everything from the treatment of hypertension to the removal of colonic polyps. It has been suggested that such an "adversary system" of presenting clinical problems be utilized routinely in teaching medicine. In this way doctors would, from the beginning of their careers, learn of the conflicts and uncertainties, rather than being doled out "the straight facts."

There are dangers to this suggested approach. To begin with, many students are depressed and frustrated by an approach that leads them to conclude that *nothing* is reliably known. In addition, there is danger of inducing the hypercritical state. To be a virtue, critique must fall somewhere between petulant querulousness and blind faith, and not deteriorate into cynical disenchantment and disengagement from life. As C. S. Lewis put it: "The only point of seeing through something is to see something through it. . . . If you see through everything, then everything is transparent. But a wholly transparent world is an invisible world. To see through all things is the same as not to see."

But there is less danger of excessive spleen than of bland intellectual oatmeal. In American medical science, it is not considered genteel to engage in blunt criticism of poor work or even fraud. Reasons given range from "It's not needed when the stuff is so blatantly bad" to "There's no point in merely destructive criticism." The English critic James Agate once pointed out, however, that whatever may be feasible in the domain of Lewis Carroll, in the world as we know it, constructiveness is possible only before an event. We ought to be able to achieve a golden mean of some sort, aiming at an atmosphere between that of a girls' school tea and the last act of *Götterdämmerung*.

A complicating bit of reality is the fact that the physician cannot avoid making decisions. Should one operate, or not? Is it appendicitis, or just a belly ache? Has the patient had a heart attack or not? What antibiotic should I prescribe for the patient's obvious meningitis while waiting for the lab reports to tell what the infecting organism is? The medical interests of the great philosopher John Locke probably contributed in no small degree to his empiricism. A scholar can be a thoroughgoing skeptic or agnostic in the confines of his study, but Locke could not afford a suspension of intellectual commitment at the bedside of the sick.

There are still other paradoxes. The pediatrician is exquisitely trained to care for critically ill, hospitalized patients, but spends the majority of his time in practice examining healthy babies and tending to trivial complaints. The internist-in-training is taught a great deal about dramatic acute illnesses, but much less about the special problems of chronic disease that will be challenging him daily in practice.

The medical student, intern, and resident usually think in terms of the hospitalized patient—a person cut off from both the stresses and the consolations of job, family, and community. The patient must eventually, however, return to the outside world. It is pointless to adjust an elderly Italian-born diabetic lady's blood sugar with great precision on a typical American hospital diet that in no way resembles what she will eat upon discharge, or to assume that a cardiac patient who can walk a hospital corridor in comfort will be able to climb the four flights to his walkup apartment.

The doctor must also respect simultaneously the general and the individual. As a scientist, he accepts as fundamental a lawfulness in natural phenomena. The respect of physicians for natural law is superimposed, however, on a necessary appreciation of variability, of richness of expression. Edith Hamilton, the famous Greek scholar, was overjoyed to learn that no one else anywhere on earth had fingerprints exactly like hers. One can listen to hundreds of chests during the pneumonia season and never hear two that sound exactly alike.

One of the most interesting contrasts is between the image of the doctor as father-priest-deity, omniscient, omnipotent, not to be disobeyed, and the fact that many patients are remarkably unwilling to follow their physician's directions and advice. The medical literature abounds with examples of this phenomenon among patients with rheumatoid arthritis and peptic ulcer, schizophrenia and urinary-tract infections. Some of these patients fail to have their prescriptions filled, others take fewer pills or more pills than were ordered. This happens even when intelligent parents are entrusted with the responsibility of getting antibiotics into their small children. Many doctors seem blithely unaware of this situation. In a survey by a Cornell team, 42 per cent of the doctors surveyed estimated that "almost all" of their patients followed their advice, and another 47 per cent estimated that three fourths do as they are told.

Doctors have contradictory desires to modify public attitudes and yet to keep the public out of scientific matters. For example, there is a tendency in the profession to sneer at the physician who makes a part-time living educating the public by writing syndicated columns or articles for news magazines or newspapers.

There is a special dilemma for physicians who wish to serve society in the larger sense, to act as citizens with special knowledge. Many laymen and doctors assume, for example, that in drafting laws on sociomedical problems legislators will systematically seek expert guidance. In fact, testimony may be remarkably haphazard or bizarre at legislative hearings dealing with medical matters, and the scientist who feels he has important facts to present had better thrust himself aggressively forward.

In interacting with members of the city, state, and national governments, the physician may quickly find himself distracted from his responsibility, either by a distaste for politicking or by the need to develop a new language if he is to talk with public figures instead of to them. The day-to-day, standard operating procedure of the scientist is inappropriate to this purpose, which requires the doctor to aim at a special kind of clarity and synthesis, making points with emphasis and economy. He also has to become reconciled to compromise and the achievable, even if this is accomplished only by fighting hard for the unattainable.

The rewards of such public performance are primarily private. While some scientists relish the power to influence public officials, or the press coverage all too easily obtained with a catchy phrase, most physicians derive little benefit from forays into public life. For academicians, even a sally into the arena of local medical societies can be painful, engendering cynicism more often than fulfillment. A brush with experienced politicians can be more traumatic.

I still recall with anger a request to testify before a Congressional committee in 1962 on the drug bill then known as H.R. 6245. After several days spent in preparing a statement, I was asked by the assistant counsel of the committee to expand it so as to include material I had previously submitted to a Senate committee. This I did. The day before my scheduled appearance he called to ask whether I would delete certain passages and include still others, which he read to me. A few of the suggestions represented minor changes in phrasing; others would have drastically altered the intent of the original statement.

It was evident that the assistant counsel did not agree with some of my sentiments. He considered them inconsistent with previous testimony. I pointed out that my views were bound to reflect the passage of time and the accumulation of information not previously available. He hung up, only to call back later in the day to explain that after discussing the matter with the chief counsel, it was apparent that my testimony "would not contribute any useful information." My appearance was canceled. Obviously what was desired was the "right kind" of testimony, not honest scientific opinion about a bill dealing with complex medical matters.

The academic physician also discovers that whereas people who agree with his actions are apt to write letters to him, those who disagree or whose toes have been trodden upon may exert pressure on his superiors at the university to castigate or silence him. Even when university officials repudiate such unsubtle muzzling attempts, the incidents are not likely to weigh in the scientist's favor when academic advancement or new posts are being considered.

But public controversy cannot be avoided. Dr. George

James discussed this matter while he was Commissioner of Health for New York City, pointing out that public health must learn to live increasingly with bitter but relevant and useful controversy. In 1906, when tuberculosis was the leading cause of death in New York City, 75 per cent of the dairy herds tributary to the local milkshed contained tuberculous cows and 10 per cent of the street samples of milk were found to be infected with live tuberculosis organisms. Pasteurization was urged as a health measure, but the dairy industry stated flatly that it could not and should not be forced to use this new technique, which would be economically ruinous and deprive millions of babies of milk because of the great increase in cost. In time, of course, the milk industry did learn how to develop pasteurization, but only because there was keen public concern and pressure for the prevention of tuberculosis and other milk-borne infections.

The enlightened physician also recognizes the need for functioning as a citizen of the world and forgoing parochial, nationalistic boundaries to health. In the 1946 preamble to the constitution of the World Health Organization, it is pointed out that:

> The health of all people is fundamental to the attainment of peace and security and is dependent upon the fullest cooperation of individuals and States.
>
> The achievement of any State in the promotion and protection of health is of value to all.
>
> Unequal development in different countries in the promotion of health and control of disease, especially communicable disease, is a common danger.

The spread of smallpox to Britain from India and Pakistan by airplane passengers, of typhoid fever to tourists in Switzerland, of resistant malaria to U.S. troops in Southeast Asia (who may spread it at home on their return) is a dramatic example of the shrinking size of our medical world and the truth of the 1946 preamble.

Physicians can play an increasingly important role in decreasing world tensions that threaten to destroy us all. There is a tradition that advances in medicine transcend political barriers and even friend-or-foe considerations in time of war. But free exchange of medical knowledge is still not a reality in all parts of the world. In 1957 the otolaryngologist Dr. Samuel Rosen of New York City demonstrated his operation to cure deafness from otosclerosis in the USSR, following which the technique was widely and effectively used in that country. But almost a decade later Rosen was forbidden by our State Department to travel to Red China on a similar mission.

It is depressing to contrast this episode with the situation in October of 1813, when Michael Faraday went to Europe with Sir Humphrey and Lady Davy. Davy's fame as a scientist had spread throughout Europe, and he was allowed to travel through France, despite the fact that England was at war with Napoleon. Davy remarked: "If two countries or governments are at war, the men of science are not. . . . That would indeed be a civil war of the worst description."

There are ways in which physicians can work even more directly to decrease the risks and horrors of war. Dr. Dimitri D. Venediktov, adviser to the USSR Permanent UN Mission in New York, has urged that doctors explain to political leaders and the public the detrimental consequences of thermonuclear and biological wars. American doctors individually and through such groups as Physicians for Social Responsibility have worked just to this purpose, testifying before Congress, lecturing to the public, visiting politicians, holding press conferences.

The entire matter of participation in warlike research has been a cause of much soul-searching among medical scientists. As a scientist, the physician may have one attitude toward the devising of techniques for poisoning a population, brainwashing the enemy, or for devising protection against such warfare. As a citizen, however, he may well wonder whether he should participate in any such research.

One of the most important contributions to be made by physicians and other scientists lies in attempting to change the fundamental political thinking of our governments. These matters are ordinarily thought to lie outside the purview of medicine—but perhaps it would not be undesirable to extend some of the rules of science to the world of politics.

We are constantly asked to make political decisions, for example, without adequate facts upon which to base a judgment. We receive third- and fourth-hand information in regard to what is going on in Europe, or Cuba, or China, rather than having multiple firsthand sources of information. It is as if one were asked to judge the Miss Universe beauty contest by utilizing the reports of chambermaids cleaning up the hotel rooms of the candidates. As Manès Sperber has written: "It is high time that those men who would interpret facts without knowing them, like eunuchs giving lessons in the art of love, should at last fall silent."

Nor does it make sense for a nation's leaders to lead a country to the brink of disaster on the basis of irrational thinking and frozen attitudes that are the political analogy of the disordered thoughts of mental illness. A provocative report in this regard was the 1964 document prepared by the Group for the Advancement of Psychiatry. It pointed out that many of the traditional stereotypes concerning the courage and manliness involved in war are psychologically questionable, and that resort to violence is apt to stem not only from anger or strength but from fear and weakness.

The report listed some psychological factors that render more difficult the achievement of nonviolent solutions to our present problems. Defense mechanisms such as denial, emotional isolation, and habituation enable people to live in the shadow of imminent nuclear annihilation without searching for ways to remove or reduce the awesome danger. We tend to be trapped by the basic human need to fit perceptions into pre-existent frames of reference. These distortions lead to stereotyped conceptions, both of oneself and of the adversary, hamper communication, lead to mutual distrust and a biased perception of what is fair and reasonable. They also provoke reciprocal behavior from the adversary, so that the mutual expectation that "the other side doesn't really want peace and can't be trusted" tends to become self-fulfilling. Such factors exert a significant pressure upon political leaders, who are caught in a conflict between the things they have to say and do to maintain their power and prestige at home, and the taking of the kinds of initiative that might lead to a lessening of tension with the adversary.

In one of the key scenes of Bertolt Brecht's *Galileo*, the aging Galileo warns that if scientists do not shoulder their social responsibilities, they become nothing but a race of inventive dwarfs. It is given to few doctors to be giants, but if there is to be a bright future for mankind—indeed if there is to be any future—the physician must modify his traditional role as servant to the sick person and take up an additional burden as servant to the sick society. The early Christians considered "Languid Indifference" one of the deadly sins; it is especially deadly today.

2

Wanted: Up-to-Date Medical Schools for a Modern World

LIKE THE DOCTOR, American medical schools present a study in paradoxes. At a time of growing apprehension about a doctor shortage, half the college students seeking admission to medical schools are being turned away. The considerable official pride in the quality of U.S. medical training contrasts vividly with appalling deficiencies in the health care provided to American citizens. The fact that most medical-school graduates intend to practice is hard to reconcile with the selection of research-oriented faculty members who scorn the "trade-school" aspects of their jobs. Doctors must deal repeatedly with the most complicated kinds of ethical, life-and-death decisions, ranging from abortion to euthanasia, but during their years in medical school there is almost no serious discussion of these matters.

Since World War II, there has been a considerable expansion of the American medical establishment. Over a dozen new schools have been started, an equal number are in the planning stages, and many of the existing schools have increased their enrollments. Whereas there were 21,000 students enrolled in 1940, there are now more than 32,000.

Despite this growth, the schools have failed to keep pace with public needs. In part, the deficiencies are traceable to an increasing preoccupation with research, stimulated by the availability of private and—especially—federal funds. Since research money represented the area where the fiscal "action" was, the medical schools have grown enormously in staff and facilities devoted to research. There has been no comparable burgeoning of nonresearch functions. As Dean William R. Willard of the University of Kentucky put it: "Most medical schools have avoided any major commitment of effort in helping to resolve the problems inherent in the delivery of health services to the people."

The fact that only about half of the students who wish to go to medical school can be accommodated suggests at first glance that medical schools have many more suitable applicants than they can handle, and that the profession or the American Medical Association maintains a monopolistic stranglehold on medical practice. Many of these students, however, are unacceptable because they have gone to poor schools or have done poorly in good schools. Other applicants are turned away because of inferior performance on medical-aptitude tests or for personality problems.

Furthermore, the schools themselves, not the AMA, determine admission policies.[1] The most famous schools have never had any problem filling their classes with promising students. Those schools that are less well known have difficulty in finding enough suitable candidates. State-supported schools

---

[1] In 1967, after years of denial, even the AMA conceded that there was a shortage of doctors. The House of Delegates recommended an "immediate and unprecedented" expansion of medical-school facilities. AMA pressures on medical schools during the depression decade of the 1930's presumably contributed to a drop in student enrollment at that time. Thereafter, AMA influence was exerted indirectly, through opposition to federal aid to medical education.

tend to discriminate against applicants whose homes are not within the confines of the state, and they wind up with less able students than do schools with unrestricted admission policies. As a result, promising candidates from some parts of the country are at a real disadvantage in seeking admission. Since the number of dropouts is also above average in schools with restricted admission policies, a deplorable waste of ability results.

In the past, even medical schools that could have expanded their classes without lowering their standards have resisted expansion because of apathy, inconvenience, cost, or lack of facilities and staff. Harvard, for example, has been turning out about the same number of doctors per year since 1930. This situation is changing in many schools, however; while there has been some foot-dragging, there is no conspiracy to hold down the number of doctors.

The total number of applicants has also been restricted by the inordinate amount of time and money required to become a physician. Young people are increasingly eager to marry early and to begin earning a living as soon as possible, and medical-school and hospital training are formidable obstacles to both goals. After college and medical school, the average specialist in internal medicine will have to put in an additional six years: two in the armed forces, one as intern, and three as resident. In some surgical specialties, it may take nine additional years after medical school before independent practice.

There is also unmistakably greater competition among the professions for bright young men today. A century ago, talented young men who wished to undertake a profession had only three choices: medicine, law, or theology. During the decades immediately after our Civil War, 28 per cent of all college graduates entered the practice of medicine. In this climate President Gilman of Johns Hopkins University observed that the medical student was likely to be "one son of the family too weak to labour on the farm, too indolent to do any exercise, too stupid for the bar and too immoral for the pulpit." Today, as many college graduates head for careers in such glamorous areas as physics, aeronautics, and big business, the proportion entering medicine has shrunk to 2 per cent.

A recent study has documented a similar human drought in Canada, where press articles and editorials had expressed concern that many qualified applicants were being rejected. About three fifths of the applications there are from Canadian citizens, one third from U.S. citizens, and the rest from overseas. The schools were asked to rate applicants as "clearly acceptable," "clearly unacceptable," or "marginal." Only 40 per cent of the Canadians were unequivocally acceptable. If one added the questionable ones, there were just about as many candidates as there were places to be filled, giving the schools no margin of choice.

While no one can prophesy with assurance who will turn out to be a good doctor, the general Canadian standard of a second-class (or B) average, preferably with no failures or "makeups," is not unreasonable.[2] Many of the applicants who applied to several schools simultaneously were graded marginal or unacceptable by all schools. Informal reports from some schools suggest that the last five or six candidates granted a place in each class are below the standards that the school has set as desirable. The study concluded that "it is erroneous to speak of a surplus of qualified applicants for the study of medicine." (If U.S. and Canadian schools, whose classes usually run between 70 and 150, suffer from a relative dearth of topnotch applicants, one must wonder about the caliber of students in certain European schools that admit classes of 600 or more.) At the same time, most medical educators would admit that *some* qualified candidates almost certainly fail to be admitted to any school.

[2] On the other hand, the University of Rochester has reported that unimpressive performance on the Medical College Admissions Test—at least when counteracted by good interviews or strong recommendations—does not presage an undistinguished medical career.

This situation is particularly serious in view of the widening "doctor gap." In 1959, the Surgeon General's Consultant Group on Medical Education warned that medical-school output was not keeping pace with the needs of the population, and that the doctor-to-population ratio had dropped since 1949.[3] Long before that, U.S. hospitals had been acutely aware of a shortage of doctors. Of some 12,000 approved internships, about 20 per cent go begging every year, despite the fact that one fifth the total number of house-staff officers are graduates of foreign medical schools. This imported contribution to U.S. medical care is even more marked in such specialties as physical medicine, pathology, and anesthesiology, where many residency programs would be crippled without foreign trainees.

In rebuttal, it has been said that the ratio of doctors to population—now close to 150 per 100,000—has actually *increased* slightly of late. This is statistical legerdemain, however. In 1964, after a conference called by the Health Resources Advisory Committee, all interns and residents, the June medical graduates, physicians with temporary foreign addresses, and others whose addresses were temporarily not known were included in the calculation of the physician-population ratio. As a result, the ratio "rose," but there were no more doctors than before—they were simply counting heads they had formerly disregarded. The ratio has been maintained only by the influx of foreign graduates, who are almost half as numerous as the graduates of our own schools.

But even if one were satisfied with the published ratios, the figures do not begin to tell the whole story. An overall ratio does not, for example, take into account physicians involved in research, administration, or other pursuits that divert them from providing medical care. Furthermore, the average for the country is as meaningless as other average figures when specific instances are being considered. The ratio of doctors to public

[3] Although this report is the one most often referred to, other analyses had come to similar conclusions about a doctor shortage as far back as 1933.

in Manhattan is close to 400 per 100,000, but this is small consolation to the inhabitants of the many small American communities that have no physician at all. (The District of Columbia has seven times as many physicians per capita as Alabama
and Mississippi.) Nor does the ratio reveal qualitative deficiencies in medical care. Almost every specialty group in the country, from clinical pharmacology to ophthalmology, radiology
to pathology, has stressed the need for more physicians trained
in its particular discipline. The number of medical-school graduates becoming so-called first-contact physicians—general
practitioners and internists—has also declined, from 55 per cent
in the first quarter of this century to 35 per cent in the last
decade.

Many doctors are faced with impossible numbers of
patients to see. I have known physicians to forsake the practice
of medicine because they cannot care adequately for the sick
in their practices. The evaluation of a new patient takes time,
as does a complication in an old case, or any patient sick enough
to be in the hospital. Such problems cannot be dealt with on
a fifteen-minute appointment schedule. An overworked doctor
does justice neither to the sick nor to himself; a British pediatrician complained of his energies being drained "by seeing too
many patients while trying to remain both human and
humane."

In addition, the population has changed in ways that affect
national needs. There are, for example, more individuals at
both extremes of the age spectrum, with the special medical
requirements of the old and the young. Medicare, Medicaid,
and the increasing national prosperity and improved economic
underpinning of medical care by prepaid health insurance have
made it possible for many people to demand medical services
they could not afford before. The poor are no longer content
to die quietly before their time.

The maternal mortality rate of nonwhites in the United
States remains a shocking reality. In 1963 there were 24 mater-

nal deaths per 100,000 live births in whites as against 98 in nonwhites. Negroes still lack equal access to hospital facilities in many areas and are often cared for by Negro physicians, who are in even shorter supply and more overworked than white physicians. Medicine and society must find more satisfactory ways of dealing both with the Negro youngster in Mississippi who did not like visiting the doctor because he resented having to go in the back door, and the woman eight and a half months pregnant who, after waiting three hours, was turned away from the prenatal clinic in New York City without seeing a doctor because the hospital did not serve the district in which she lived.

Patients in need of psychiatric help are more and more restive at having to choose between an expensive psychiatrist and inadequately staffed psychiatric clinics with long waiting lists. Newspaper and magazine accounts of advances in diagnosis and therapy distress readers who learn that they must go without the life-saving services of an intensive-coronary-care unit, or of a kidney-dialysis facility, simply because their local hospital does not provide such services. The chronically ill are no longer resigned to a humiliating deterioration at home, in dismal "hospitals for incurables," or in fourth-rate nursing facilities. The medical schools must, therefore, turn out more doctors. The standard approaches have been to increase the size of medical-school classes and to start new schools, but neither principle has been applied with sufficient vigor. A third approach would be to decrease the number of dropouts from medical school. If each school could salvage one student per year from this group, the effect would be equivalent to starting a new average-sized medical school.

What do we know about these dropouts? They average 10 per cent of the entering class, a low figure compared to those for nursing, law, and engineering schools, where almost half the students fail to graduate. But this mean hides the fact that dropout rates range from a few per cent to about 20. Studies by the Association of American Medical Colleges have shown that schools with low attrition rates have bigger budgets,[4] more out-of-state students, and greater motivation and higher achievement-test scores among those gaining admission.

About half the dropouts leave for nonacademic reasons, and some of these might conceivably be retained with more financial aid and psychiatric counseling. One cannot but wonder, however, whether better selection is not feasible. While simple predictive tests are not as yet available, it should at least be possible to upgrade selections by eliminating the geographical restrictions extant in many schools, which hurt both the good out-of-state student and the school.

Should not medical students be treated as a national resource rather than a local one? If so, the obvious step is to institute a national matching program for college students similar to that used to match senior medical students and approved internships. A senior medical student now applies to any number of hospitals, but the final assignment is determined strictly by the mutual attraction of hospital and intern candidate. If a student's top preference is a hospital that has him on its top list of potential interns, the computer stops there. If not, the procedure continues until all the candidates—actually a few end up unmatched—are assigned to the most desired job available to them, on a national basis. A similar scheme for admission to medical schools should work equally well, decreasing the chances of poorly qualified candidates and thus cutting down on dropouts.

The best of the present students are superb: the semifinalists for National Merit Scholarships since 1957 have been analyzed as to career choices, and medicine is second only to theoretical physics in attracting such students. But most places in medical school are not filled with Merit finalists and some

---

[4] This fact is cited by those who argue that federal research funds have enabled new faculty members to be hired and have thus importantly helped medical education.

are filled with only average students—is there an untapped pool of excellent candidates somewhere?

One almost certainly exists in the talented youngsters in our "lower social classes," a term that sounds as if it ought to be outdated but isn't. About 10 per cent of medical students come from the bottom half of our socioeconomic ladder. This partly reflects the decreased tendency of such students even to begin college, but the longer and more expensive the road to a career the more serious are the obstacles. This belief is bolstered by the evidence that schools with lower tuition rates attract more of the economically deprived students. A national program that effectively upgraded the interest of such students in advanced education of any sort and made education financially possible would undoubtedly pay dividends to the health sciences. For these candidates, however, the aid must be virtually total—loans have to be repaid, and large debts are likely to discourage a needy student.

Many of our present medical students also have problems in making ends meet, and serious debts are frequently incurred before graduation. Nor does the M.D. degree mark the end of the struggle. Even the intern averages only $3,800 per year, with another $100 when he becomes a resident.[5] For a married doctor with a wife and family, such an income is grossly inadequate. The new federal bill providing scholarship aid to medical schools should help considerably, but medical training still is not as well supported by unrefundable aid as is Ph.D. training in the arts and sciences.

The Negro student has a special problem. The rare highly qualified Negro from a good university probably has an edge over equally qualified white students, since most medical-school deans would gleefully enroll such a prospect. But what of the more typical Negro from a second-rate Southern college? Such a candidate would not get into most medical schools. (It is

[5] These figures are for 1966–7. Incomes are being increased in many places, although still not enough.

argued that if he did, he would probably be frustrated by his performance or flunk out.) He does have a better chance to enter one of the Negro medical schools, but these institutions have for years suffered from inadequate financial support and from staffs that are, with a few exceptions, less than distinguished.

As one professor of medicine from a prominent Eastern school said, "Should we have Negro schools that are in trouble and will continue to be in trouble? I personally think it would be a good thing, at least for the next twenty or thirty years, to have Negro medical schools of excellence. But at present, these schools are compelled to remain second-rate. They're told by the government and by foundations that they don't have a good enough program for long-term support, but how do you get a good enough program if you don't have money to begin with?"

Women also have special difficulties in pursuing a medical career. Although the percentage of women medical students has almost doubled since 1950, the United States still has one of the lowest percentages of women entering medicine among the world's nations. Our 9.1 per cent is on a par with the figure for Spain, where the duenna-monitored, cloistered life has been traditional for women of the upper classes. In the United Kingdom, 25 per cent of the medical students are now women, in Bulgaria and Yugoslavia 30 per cent, and in Russia about 75 per cent. In Thailand it is alleged that a ceiling of 25 per cent had to be established when the figure reached 44 per cent in 1949 and the better academic records of the girls inspired fears that medicine would become a feminine profession.

The participation of American women in medicine is limited by a variety of factors. To begin with, it is difficult to pursue a medical career and motherhood simultaneously. More women than men drop out of medical school and less of them stay in full-time medical jobs. Medical training is not flexible enough to dovetail with pregnancy and childrearing. Once she is an intern, a young doctor-mother cannot work twenty-four hours on and twenty-four hours off unless the larger medical centers establish crèches, nurseries, and kindergartens where she would be willing to leave her youngster, and she may still feel she is neglecting the child.

Once in medical school, some disturbing changes occur in medical students. There is evidence of a decline of idealism and a rise in cynicism or emotional detachment as the medical student progresses toward his M.D. degree. Two researchers at the University of Kansas found that students enter school believing the practice of medicine to be a wonderful thing that will allow them to devote their lives to the service of mankind. They further believe that medicine is made up of a great body of hard facts, which need only to be mastered in order for a man to become a good doctor. The disillusionment begins quickly, when the students learn that the first year or two is just like college, with discussion of medical care and patients nowhere in sight. The subject matter—which may be taught less well than similar subjects were at college—seems almost irrelevant to the practice of medicine.

Even worse is the realization that there is more to medicine than can possibly be learned by one man. There is a temptation to believe that this is a relatively new problem, but Dr. Jacob Bigelow of Harvard said in 1850:

> In modern times the constituent branches of medical science are so expanded that they cannot be acquired by any physician in a lifetime and still less by a student in his pupilage. The same is true even of many individual branches. It is not therefore to be concluded that "a scheme of scientific instruction should embrace the whole science and no part should be omitted," nor that "a well digested plan of lecture embrace all that is to be known and taught." Medical science has at this day become so unwieldy and contains so much that is necessary, at least to beginners, that the attempt to explain to stu-

dents the whole is likely to involve the result of their learning but little.

The student then substitutes a more attainable goal—the ability to learn what the faculty expects him to learn, regardless of whether he may consider it important. Eventually, when the student does get to deal with patients, it is often to learn a medical problem rather than to help a sick person. He often has little responsibility in the care of the patient and must resign himself to vicarious participation in the dramatic and dangerous clinical situations that he believes to be the core of medical practice. Problems that might evoke idealistic postures are rarely discussed. Perhaps medical students put idealism aside only temporarily in favor of the reality of getting through school, but one wonders whether the displacement is not often a permanent one.

I still remember with disappointment the lack of adequate discussion, among my medical colleagues and students, of the death of Norman Morrison, the local Quaker who burned himself alive outside the Pentagon on November 2, 1965. Even a wise professor of psychiatry from another university with whom I spent the morning after the event automatically assumed that such a gesture could only be the senseless act of a deranged mind.

Those of us who knew Morrison even slightly, however, could not accept such a facile explanation. As one of his friends put it, Morrison was abnormal in the sense that we live in a society where it is normal for human beings to drop bombs on other human beings, or to spend 50 per cent of the tax dollar on war, or to give children war toys for Christmas. By those criteria, Morrison was highly, proudly abnormal.

But the point here is that so devastating a form of human behavior as suicide is barely touched upon within the medical school. It is easy to guess why most people dismissed the burning as an insane act. Many people have no deep feelings about anything, let alone a willingness to give up their lives for some ideal or goal. It is more comfortable for them to reject the purposeful giving up of life for a cause than to admit to their consciousness the possibility of such an act. The result is to demean the unselfish, sacrificial act with reflex clichés. Contrast, instead, the last words of a leader of the German opposition to Hitler: "The worth of a man is certain only if he is prepared to sacrifice his life to his convictions."

Many educators are concerned about the undesirable consequences of the type of medical curriculum prevalent in our schools. They see a need for new curricula that will be both richer and more relevant to the student's needs. Such revision is not a simple matter—the neurosurgeon Harry Cushing once said that to change a medical-school curriculum was harder than moving a graveyard—but the wheels of change are in motion.

Abraham White, a biochemist who helped develop the medical schools at UCLA and Yeshiva, is one of a growing number who repudiate the notion that the curriculum of a school is the property of its individual departments, organized for their convenience. He asks that the curriculum be designed for, and given back to, the students, and reminds the faculty that the goal of the student is to become a physician. Peter V. Lee, of the University of Southern California, has expressed similar sentiments and recommends the creation of curricula that are fully patient-oriented from the beginning. He argues that for physicians the basic medical sciences as disciplines have no meaning unless they have relevance to human beings and human illness.

But this revision alone is not sufficient. It must be coupled with increased flexibility. The post-Flexner[6] revolution in medical education evolved a relatively Procrustean format involving

[6] Abraham Flexner's *Medical Education in the United States and Canada*, published in 1910, led to the abolition of diploma mills and other substandard schools.

two related assumptions that are no longer valid: that medical students are a relatively homogeneous lot, and that they should all be trained in the same way.

Today's students come to medical school with college backgrounds that differ tremendously. Some have had a heavy dose of science courses, others very little. Some have had superb training in modern biology that has anticipated (if not outdone) much of the program they are required to sit through during their first year in medical school, while others are inadequately prepared.

The career goals of the medical students are also vastly different. A student headed for practice hardly needs the same type of training as one headed for research. Indeed, the researcher who plans to spend his life in the laboratory and the researcher who is headed for clinical investigation need not be exposed to exactly the same things, any more than the psychiatrist and the orthopedic surgeon need identical training.

Students also differ in their response to different pedagogic methods. Some thrive on didactic lectures, others detest them. Some find teaching machines acceptable and efficient, others get inspiration from small group Socratic discussion. (And for some, the best advice for the faculty is to stand back out of their way.)

Whether most medical schools can afford or attain the high degree of flexibility suggested by the above considerations is another matter, but the faults of the frozen curriculum seem clear. Good graduate programs leading to the Ph.D. are tailor-made—why not for the M.D.?

Medical schools face another dilemma in choosing between the teaching of facts and the teaching of principles. There are more and more bits of information waiting to be taught, and while today's facts may be tomorrow's nonsense, it is impossible to practice medicine without mastering a certain body of knowledge and technology. The problem lies in deciding what to teach and how to avoid teaching it in a manner one educator has compared to the stuffing of Strasbourg geese

—cramming it down the throats of students who have no alternative but to swallow obediently with a minimum of struggle.

There must be a balance of some kind between detail and principle, but the M.D. candidate must also acquire critique and the ability to continue his education after the formal training years so that he may continue to function effectively throughout his career. One popular suggestion is to allow more free time in the curriculum, so as to force the student to assume responsibility for his own maturation. This poses another dilemma: how can the student have more free time when there is so much more each year to cover?[7]

Regrettably, the laudable desire to increase the percentage of elective time has become almost synonymous, in some schools, with the participation of medical students in research. Admirable as this may be for some, it is highly questionable as a routine device for most students. Lewis Thomas, dean at New York University, has said that the opportunity to work in a research lab is a privilege that no more than 25 per cent of the student body either merits or wants.

Pushing students into unwanted and unneeded research activity are two potent forces. The first is the research-suffused atmosphere in many schools, which makes a student feel like a second-class citizen if he doesn't show an interest in research, with potential penalties in the form of less than enthusiastic recommendations for internship. (A student who is an incompetent physician may get a sterling letter of support from a professor whom he assisted capably on a research project.) The second is the availability of funds to support students who sign up for research. These awards are in fact only thinly disguised subsidies, and it would be far better if federal and other funds for this purpose could be honestly split up among all medical students requiring financial aid.

No matter how much time is allocated to student initia-

---

[7] It has been argued that eventually science acquires great principles and laws that substitute the general for the specific and free man from the tyranny of unrelated facts, but that happy day is not yet at hand for medicine.

tive, however, there remains the question of the core curriculum. What minimum should be required of every medical student? If a man is to receive the M.D. degree, with its legal implication that the holder may obtain a license to care for the sick, what must he have shown himself capable of? Certainly anyone who claims to be a physician must be able to take a proper medical history and perform a competent physical examination. (This statement is true despite the fact that most doctors get through medical school without ever having another doctor watch them do a complete physical examination from beginning to end.) It may be argued, quite reasonably, that a medical student headed for laboratory research has no need to master even the core curriculum, but then there seems little reason for such a person to acquire an M.D. Why not give him the older and more traditional Ph.D.?

The principle of a core curriculum is important also because it implies another principle: a responsible overseeing of the total content of the curriculum by some faculty committee, a mechanism for seeing to it that important matters are not omitted because each department assumes that somebody else will teach them.There is a strong tradition in many schools that each department may teach what it considers appropriate. This philosophy is attractive to a faculty that treasures its independence, but may result in the student hearing about protein synthesis five or six different times, while the proper use of sedatives and tranquilizers is not even covered once.

For training modern doctors, the present departmental structure is archaic. Medical schools have been divided into departments for reasons of history and for convenience, originally at a time when the various medical sciences were evolving distinctly and separately. With the inevitable segmentation of knowledge, each segment came under the jurisdiction of an individual department, with little or no relationship or communication between departments.

For the years immediately before and after the First World

War, such a structure functioned well enough, and was a great improvement over the pre-Flexner schools. Since World War II, however, the distinctions between departments have blurred. Today it is often difficult to tell a pharmacologist from a biochemist, a microbiologist from a geneticist. The student is all too aware of the discrepancy between the background of a teacher and the course he is assigned to teach. Either strict departmental teaching tends to reflect less what is supposed to be taught than the department's research interests or the department becomes a booking agency, calling on radiologists or surgeons to teach anatomy, or clinical specialists to teach pharmacology or microbiology.

Although departmental barriers in respect to teaching should be destroyed, cohesive departments for the coordination of research and the training of research scientists should be maintained. These activities are legitimate functions, and are indeed necessary to keep the school intellectually alive, but they are separate from the teaching of medical students. The school must foster research, but it cannot tolerate educational anarchy.

Medical students should also be able to elect exposure to the specialized wares offered by a top-notch faculty with multiple research interests. A teacher should teach students about the things that he knows best and that really excite him—but not every student. I believe that many a medical-school professor would prefer talking to a handful of students really eager to hear what he has to say about a specialized topic dear to his heart to lecturing on the same topic to a large captive audience, two fifths of which is asleep and another two fifths in acute intellectual pain.

Providing a rich intellectual smorgasbord of electives seems the only way of presenting to students the possible careers open to a medical man. There are many areas important for society but now relatively neglected, including public health, preventive medicine, community medicine, medical history, medical economics, most of the surgical specialties, anesthesiology, radiology, and clinical pharmacology. These cannot all be taught, unless it is done so superficially as to defeat the purpose, despite the fact that each specialty group, given the chance, will demand its place, no matter how small, and its time, no matter how brief, in the curricular sun. Yet no specialty can be allowed to atrophy for total lack of exposure.

The student will not, however, accept as important what the faculty does not consider important. If the costs of a battery of diagnostic tests or of hospitalization are never discussed at the bedside by professors of medicine, it will do little good to have an elective course in medical economics. If the risks of a liver or kidney biopsy are not taken up when such a procedure is contemplated, there is almost no point to a theoretical discussion of medical ethics in a seminar course.

It is vital for medical schools to welcome the state of flux and accept change as both desirable and unavoidable. The "facts" of medicine change daily, our society is rapidly changing—how can the schools remain static? When it comes to the specific changes to be wrought in medical education, there is much disagreement, a healthy sign in a field where no one has a pipeline to eternal truth and where there is great need for experimentation.

One set of experiments allows students to save one or more years of time in their pursuit of the M.D. degree. At Johns Hopkins, selected students are admitted after two years of college into a five-year plan, thus allowing the M.D. to be acquired seven years after completing high school rather than the usual eight. Some few students are also allowed to bypass the free elective quarters offered each of the last four years and thus save an additional year. Although the curriculum change was originally touted as one that would save time and money for medical students, the major impact of the change has been to provide more opportunity for independent study and research, the not unmixed blessing discussed earlier. What would have been in some ways the most startling innovation—the use of the last year as an internship year, thus bringing the intern training of all Hopkins graduates under the jurisdiction of the university—was never put into effect because several department heads were unwilling to scrap the traditional intern-residency program.

Two other programs that provide acceleration are the six-year curricula at Boston University and Northwestern University. Both provide an intensive two-year premedical course designed for selected high-school graduates, followed by the traditional four-year medical curriculum. Selection for medical school must thus be made earlier than is customary, and the implication is that in terms of preparation for medicine—at least at the scientific course level—two well-planned years will do instead of four.

Another interesting experiment was recently begun at Duke University. Its most unusual feature is early career differentiation. Every student is exposed to a core of preclinical medical sciences followed by an all-purpose core patient-centered clerkship. In the third and fourth years the student and his preceptors tailor-make his program, aiming for learning in depth and more tutorial training. Roughly half the time is to be devoted to preclinical sciences and half to clinical medicine. The man headed for general practice might use his last year to acquire special knowledge about skin diseases, for example, and the future surgeon might concentrate on non-surgical fields, such as internal medicine, since he will get an abundance of surgical training during his residency. The Duke faculty hopes that the plan will "provide flexibility in place of rigidity; experience in depth for superficial exposure to material; critical evaluation for rote learning; individual experience for mass indoctrination . . ."—a devastating indictment of traditional teaching.

A potentially exciting program was planned for the new Mount Sinai Medical School in New York City. This school, unlike most others, began with no parent university and intended to create its own faculty at all levels. Its sponsors hoped to turn this seeming disadvantage to advantage by creating a new type of university—a health-science-oriented and specialized institution of higher learning, consisting of a medical school, a strong teaching hospital, and graduate schools of biologic sciences, physical sciences, and "human studies" relevant to health care, with scholars in psychology, philosophy, history, economics, sociology, and other fields in residence on the health-science campus. Recently, the school has become affiliated with the University of the City of New York, and it is not clear how this will affect the original plans.

It is often assumed that a medical school must be affiliated with a university to be first-rate, either because the affiliation provides a better-rounded training to the medical student, or because it improves the research establishment, or because it achieves economies and higher quality of service by pooling library, computer, and other facilities. Only a dozen or so of the nation's medical schools lack university affiliation. But only half the affiliated schools are geographically close to the university campus, and some are hundreds of miles away. In few of them does the undergraduate school or the nonmedical graduate program affect the life of the medical student. The integration of medical schools and universities is very much like racial integration—important, but rarely achieved.

The earliest example of the new curricula was established at Western Reserve University in 1952, when a new dean and many new department heads determined to cross departmental lines and establish interdisciplinary teaching, family clinics, early patient contacts, and other innovations that seem less controversial now than they did then. The results have been generally pleasing to the faculty and students. The Western Reserve program has helped to free medical educators from the bonds of conformity, although it may seem old-fashioned today when compared to some of the newest plans.

It is not just the curricula of medical schools that need revision. Their faculties also require reappraisal, as well as the very phenomenon of teaching itself. Dr. T. C. King has complained that teachers of medicine and those responsible for curriculum planning and program evaluation, despite exceptional skills as research scientists, often bring no professional educational skill to their complex tasks as teachers and administrators:

> The pattern of medical school teacher selection, particularly when it comes to department chairmen, is analogous to the professional football coach who signs a quarterback to a long term contract on the basis of the athlete's record as an exceptional 400 yard breaststroke swimmer. Since he is such a good swimmer, there is no real need to watch him play football before handing him the responsibility for guiding the football team nor is there even any reason to expect him to acquire some training in that sport.

While requiring education courses for medical-school teachers seems questionable, in view of the poor quality of many professional schools of education and the tenuous relationship between formal education training and teaching ability, it is certainly a good idea to have good teachers. And it is not difficult to judge a good teacher if he has had a chance at teaching.[8]

A few years ago a committee was chosen to select a new head of surgery at a medical school that prides itself on training research doctors. One of the committee members, a world-famous biochemist, made the remarkable assertion that the first requirement for the job was that the candidate should be a capable biochemist. When one considers that the professor of surgery must be responsible for the quality of the surgery practiced on his service and the quality of the surgical training

---

[8] Dr. David Seegal has suggested that we begin by training every medical student to be an effective teacher, since his career will inevitably require this of him.

available to the surgical interns and residents on his staff, the fatuousness of this remark is appalling. One wonders whether biochemists really wish to have their infected gallbladders removed by other biochemists!

In 1965 Dr. Carl A. Moyer, just before resigning his post as head of surgery at Washington University at St. Louis, made the following statement to the graduating class there:

> Professors in medical schools are evidently somewhat repelled by [medical students], judging from the increasing infrequency with which students are taught by senior professors. Seemingly, today the surest way to a chair on a medical school faculty is to isolate oneself from teaching chores and become apprenticed to a scientist in a place such as the National Institutes of Health, where there are no medical students on whom one needs to waste one's precious climbing time.

Hovering balefully over the medical-school scene today is the pathetic delusion that molecular biology, the study of the inner workings of the cell, will somehow bring the answers to all the medical problems facing mankind. One even hears basic-science professors prophesying the practice of medicine at the molecular level. This philosophy will work no better in the twentieth century than it did two millennia ago when it was called "atomism" instead of "reductionism"—is it possible that proponents of molecular medicine are uninfluenced by such nonmolecular things as history and philosophy?

It is perhaps not surprising that devotees of molecular biology should downgrade curricular concern with medical economics, community medicine, rehabilitation, medical planning, and administration. Perspective on the broad sweep of human society is the antithesis of focusing on a cell fragment under an electron microscope; but the cracking of the genetic code, exciting as it is, will not comfort a latter-day Jeremiah crying: "Is there no balm in Gilead? Is there no physician there?"

It is both a pity and a waste that medical-school faculties have in many instances pridefully moved away from the study of man and his individual and social problems, in the mistaken notion that there is something intrinsically nobler and more important about cellular or subcellular research. Dr. William B. Castle, professor of medicine at Harvard, spoke to this point on receiving the Kober Medal of the Association of American Physicians in 1962. He asked that research not be judged in proportion to the complexity of the technique involved or inversely to the size of the object investigated. In his view, the study of the patient, including all aspects of his disease and of its relation to his physical and cultural environment, is the "basic" research area appropriate for the physician.

It would be equally shortsighted to insist on a ban on cellular research in medical schools, although Dr. John H. Gibbon, Jr., head of surgery at Jefferson Medical School in Philadelphia, has gone so far as to say that "the Ph.D. scientist has no place in a medical school, teaching medical students. Medical students should be taught by men and women . . . who have taken care of patients themselves and know what the student is going to face when he goes out into the world." (Dr. Gibbon admitted that his theories are "way out of line" with current practice but remarked: "I'm getting close to retirement and can afford to say what I think.")

There is, rather, a compelling need to integrate the "new biology" so rapidly evolving at the basic-science level into the teaching of medicine. Dr. Robert R. Wagner, professor of microbiology at the University of Virginia, has predicted that failure to bridge the widening gap between biology and medicine will result in the relegation of medicine to a subservient technology that contributes little to scientific knowledge and is plagued by second-rate teaching and students and by a lack of communication between the physician and the biomedical scientist. Wagner's predictions may be excessively gloomy, but the issues are not imaginary.

While it is customary to voice concern about the qualitative makeup of the faculty, the sheer numbers of faculty usually come in for less discussion, despite the fact that studies of twenty-eight medical schools have shown high faculty-student ratios to be happily correlated with the ability and attitudes of the students. This point is likely to become increasingly discussed as pressure on the medical schools to provide more service to the public grows.

President Johnson's Administration has de-emphasized research while increasing federal support for health-service facilities, the most dramatic push in this latter direction being the founding of the heart disease–cancer–stroke regional centers. At the same time, the public has begun its own squeeze by using hospital emergency rooms increasingly in place of visits to doctors' offices. Some hospitals have had a 500 per cent increase in emergency-room traffic since World War II, with a change in the nature of the visits from true emergencies to a more or less representative cross section of complaints, many of them chronic in nature.

Since the present complement of clinicians in university departments is already overworked, the new pressures require the creation of new jobs. One suggestion is that universities appoint additional physicians whose major, if not sole, responsibility will be the organization of patient services. If the universities are also to expand their teaching responsibilities for postgraduate training, someone will have to shoulder those new tasks as well. Some fear, however, that these new appointees would be granted less than full citizenship in the academic community, with serious divisive effects on both the faculty and the curriculum.

It is exciting to consider the possible gains to the country of rethinking medical education at a national level, including not only the more effective utilization of student talent but also the qualitative and quantitative needs for physicians in different parts of the country. The medical needs of isolated areas is a case in point. At present, cities have a relative over-abundance of physicians while small communities are doctor-poor. The problem is in part a matter of logistics, and the intelligent use of modern transportation could certainly improve the health care of patients requiring specialized diagnostic or therapeutic skills unavailable locally but available at nearby centers.

Yet there remains a need for doctors to provide the thousand and one services that are required of a doctor in rural practice and that cannot be conveniently or economically handled by bundling up everyone with a medical problem and driving or flying him to the nearest center. Luring good doctors to rural areas is difficult. The financial rewards are minimal, the life is likely to be restricted culturally and educationally for wife and children, and the intellectual breath of life that comes from contact with a teaching hospital is usually missing. Remedies for these various deficiencies are not readily apparent.

At least two states have tried to ease the problem by granting students loans that are canceled when the student agrees to service a "medical poverty pocket" for a specified period after graduation. The program in Florida has been going long enough to permit preliminary assessments of its efficiency. Dr. Homer L. Pearson, Jr., director of the Florida Board of Medical Examiners, has reported that the idea is not working very well. Despite $1,000 loans to students for each year of school and two years of residency training, hardly any of the students seem to end up in small towns—they prefer to pay back the loans.

The Sears Roebuck Foundation has done better with a more carefully thought-out plan: a community that passes an economic test showing that a doctor can expect to net at least $15,000 a year is then helped to construct a modern medical building. Sears provides about $5,000 to $7,000 worth of expert guidance and technical know-how, and the town raises

$40,000 via a nonprofit corporation that sells shares, making the people in the community part owners of the clinic. Since 1958, the program, conducted in cooperation with the AMA, has placed 171 doctors in small communities, and 120 of these have stayed on.

Obviously, the universities must redefine their role in America's health future. An expansion of their commitment to medical care poses very real hazards. The size and budget of the medical school already elicit hostility in other parts of the university. There is also the danger that academic pursuits—the cherished ivory-tower scholasticism—may suffer if the medical school becomes overly committed to service functions.

While sympathetic to these anxieties, I believe that those who foresee in increased university commitments a destruction of the fundamental purpose of the university are out of step with history. The concept of a sequestered society of scholars and students, poring over obscure manuscripts and serving as trustees for the preservation of knowledge, died a long time ago, if indeed it ever existed. The university of today interacts increasingly with the outside world, often to the benefit of both. University architects are consulted on the building of houses and skyscrapers; university engineers advise industry; university physicians advise on space travel, atmospheric pollution, FDA decisions, Congressional appropriations and legislation. Should we reverse this trend, and remove from public service the most important supply of scientists qualified to advise and act, and the least fettered group in terms of freedom of expression, that can be found?

Furthermore, the university will be rewarded in ways that are closely related to more traditional concepts of university function. One can visualize a host of research problems emerging from an increasing interface between "town and gown," problems of greatest importance begging for research in depth. How can we increase the scientific nature, the precision, the objectivity of clinical data, of history-taking, of physical examinations, of diagnostic logic? How can we tailor drugs to patients' needs and avoid trial-and-error judgments? How can we increase the efficiency and integration of health services? What duties can nonphysicians handle effectively, thus freeing doctors for more complex medical problems? These are all legitimate subjects for inquiry by a medical school.

The university's job is to maintain an appropriate set of priorities. No school can tackle all the health problems requiring attention and do justice to them, and no school can afford to lose sight of the fundamental goal of scholarly, "unapplied" research. It may be, for example, that a school can legitimately and effectively do research in the delivery of health care even though it would be disastrous for it to commit itself to providing comprehensive health care to all members of a community. Such issues will be passionately discussed in the next decade, as the schools and the public search painfully for the right solutions to their mutual problems.

3

Have Your Doctor Checked Once a Year

E VERYONE WANTS a good doctor. Every doctor wants to be a good physician. It is thus extremely disturbing to both patients and doctors to suggest that physicians may be inept, or may become incompetent by failing to keep up with advances in medicine. Many patients assume that anything they hear about inadequacies in medical practice cannot possibly apply to their own physicians, just as it is usually that other doctor down the street who has the flashy new Cadillac, is impersonal, and is only a money-grubbing businessman at heart.

Physicians handle this same problem in different ways. One is to deny that there are any serious deficiencies in medical care. Another is to deny that one can evaluate quality in medical practice. A third is to maintain that the profession already polices its own members, and that the public is well protected by current practices. It is the purpose of this chapter to examine both public and professional attitudes and see how much truth there is in them.

We might consider first whether the public is able to evaluate medical competence. How do patients pick doctors, for example? Such data as are available suggest that many patients depend largely on casual word-of-mouth recommendations from friends or relatives, and on such easily ascertainable criteria as accessibility, bedside manner, ethnic background, and cost of services. Some of these criteria make good sense. A doctor whose services are readily available when and where they are needed is better for both the psychological and the physical well-being of the patient. Given two equally competent physicians, the one who communicates better with the patient and makes the patient feel more at ease will do the better job. The man who prefers an older doctor or the woman who desires a female physician for gynecologic complaints will not settle for a young male graduate, no matter how well trained he is. The sick person searching for an authoritarian figure who knows everything and never seems to have a doubt will be unhappy with a physician who honestly discusses his ignorance, and patients who wish to participate more fully in the patient-doctor relationship and who wish to know how certain or uncertain a doctor is at every step of the way will not tolerate a "father-knows-best" physician.

There are a few rough rules of thumb that may serve patients well. The fact that a doctor has board certification in a given specialty indicates at least a minimal amount of hospital training, as well as the ability to pass stiff oral and written examinations devised by fellow specialists. Many doctors fail these examinations, and there is a far from perfect correlation between the ability to practice medicine or surgery and the ability to pass the examinations, but there are few medical experts who do not believe that board-qualified specialists are on the average more competent than those who lack such certification. (Most doctors also use specialists for illnesses in their own family, a clear evidence of their own feelings in the matter.) When asked for advice by a distant friend or relative, I have often been able to do nothing better than to look in the AMA directory and find the name of a nearby board-certified internist or surgeon.

If a doctor is affiliated with a hospital that has teaching ties with a university it is generally a point in his favor, but affiliation with other types of hospitals is not very meaningful, since few doctors lack hospital privileges somewhere.[1] Physicians who practice in a group are often a better bet than those who do not, if only because they keep track of each other's mistakes and a patient is more likely to be seen by a consultant if he has special complaints that are beyond the competence of the physician first consulted.

There are also rough rules in picking hospitals. Hospitals affiliated with a medical school are on the average better than those that are not. Hospitals with a full complement of interns and residents generally are better than other hospitals. Most physicians send their own families to hospitals that have more than 200 beds and are of the voluntary, nonprofit, accredited type.

Ideally, the public would itself be able to gauge professional competence. A truly competitive system requires consumers who can judge quality of performance. If consumers in medicine were aware of a physician's inadequacies, the poor practitioner would be forced out, or at least would fare less well. Litigation for malpractice provides a potential check on the physician, but it is an inefficient way of monitoring medical competence. Most mistakes of physicians are unrecognized, and patients are more interested in good medical care than in recompense for bad medical care.

Patients unquestionably know more about medicine than they did a few decades ago, even if they cannot yet function effectively as a consumer force. The mass-communications media spend a great deal of time and effort in covering problems of health. Doctors are ambivalent, however, about this

---

[1] This generalization applies less well to Negro physicians in some parts of the country.

aspect of public education. As Sir William Haley, editor of the *Times* of London, pointed out, leaders of the profession are in principle in favor of "responsible" discussions of medical information and controversies, but they are often likely to restrict the definition of "responsible" so severely as to inhibit most public debate of medical matters. To be sure, the profession has some legitimate worries, such as raising false hopes or decreasing public confidence. Yet those who believe in the benefits of an enlightened society must grant the ordinary man the right to know the truth as well as the opportunity to understand it.

The public must be educated, but at the same time public demands for drugs that have been prematurely publicized must be avoided. The overenthusiastic surgeon who conducts press conferences before each new untried bit of dramatic organ replacement must be discouraged. We should be able to discuss publicly the possibility of an epidemic of smallpox, but must not disturb the population and create chaos for the local authorities who must cope with the demand for vaccination. Thus there is a delicate balance between helpful and harmful public information.

One answer lies in better reporting. We cannot prevent the coverage of sensational but ill-advised medical announcements, but with responsible and capable medical reporting, either by talented lay journalists or by scientists willing to engage in popular writing, such problems can be minimized. There is a clear trend toward a higher quality of science reporting in the United States and elsewhere, primarily in the larger publications, but the majority of newspapers cannot afford to maintain a staff capable of handling local scientific and medical announcements quickly and in depth.

Some excellent medical journalism is written by qualified physicians, but many of them are discouraged by the low opinion of such activity held by their peers. This is difficult to understand, since the profession stands to benefit greatly from general medical reporting by physicians both competent in their fields and able to write a simple declarative sentence. It would be interesting to see how regularly scheduled radio or television programs[2] aimed at covering medical news in this way might fill the gap. A network approach to medical reporting could mobilize scientific talent for a balanced presentation much more effectively than could local stations.

The medical profession and hospital administrators must reconcile themselves to the need of news media for headlines, compression of data, and timing of news items, as well as the need to entertain the public, but the responsible reporter will still carefully check primary sources and may even improve rapport with scientific informants by confirming stories before they are filed. This routine should be the goal, not the ridiculously constricting rules that have at times been proposed by the medical profession. One suggested press-relation code actually proposed that "the physician first obtain assurance from the reporter that the story will not be published until the story is reviewed by the Chairman of the Public Relations Board of the Medical Society or his designate to be certain no violations are found, and the Chairman of the Public Relations Board will recommend changes which will serve to protect the physician against charges of violating these principles. It is earnestly hoped that the reporter will honor the assurance given the physician, thereby protecting him (the physician) against disciplinary actions and at the same time assisting the medical profession to maintain the standards of ethics." As one reporter commented, he hoped that someday there would be a code that would allow a journalist to go into the operating room and pick up a scalpel anytime he did not like the way doctors were doing things.

In 1965, the respected British medical periodical *The Lancet* said that the time had come for an airing of the issues raised by eye infections at a Birmingham hospital during the

[2] This idea has been suggested by Eliot Frankel of NBC.

previous year, as a result of which six patients each lost the sight of an eye. It took more than a year after the last incident for the Birmingham Regional Hospital Board and the Dudley Road Hospital Management Committee to issue a cautious statement on the infections and to promise a detailed report in a medical journal. Clearly mistakes had been made in regard to sterilizing, distributing, and storing fluids used in eye surgery. (Dangerous bacteria that can cause eye infections will actually grow in certain disinfectants, unless special precautions for sterilization are taken.)

One of the arguments for hushing up such problems is that the public might lose confidence in physicians or hospitals. The editorial pointed out, however, that a serious rail, air, or sea accident leads to inquiries, publication of the findings, and compensation for the victims, without destroying public confidence in the safety of trains, planes, and ships. The difference between such accidents and those in the hospital is that public accidents cannot usually be hidden, whereas those in the hospital can be and often are. The article concluded: "We are ill-served by the present widely held belief that doctors cover up for each other and for their hospitals in a way which takes too little account of the true interests of our patients and others."

Scientists are often oblivious to their own best interests in the matter of public education. Few researchers were involved in attempts to improve animal care in laboratories by creative legislation. They did ultimately respond in a defensive way to legislative propositions that were foolish and overly restrictive. In fact, the eventual legislation was generally reasonable and will probably work to the best interests of the scientists as well as of the animals. It is no secret that animal care has been, and is, far from ideal in many academic laboratories. This has at times resulted in research on animals that were infected or inadequately nourished, and the improvement of animal care should improve the quality of research.

This is not to deny the ridiculous nature of some of the

proposals made by animal lovers. Some wanted a trained physician-anesthetist to be present every time an animal of any size was subjected to surgery. Such a restriction would not only almost eliminate animal research, but would demand for animals a service considered unnecessary for humans, who throughout the world are often given anesthesia by competent and well-trained nurses. Even in the final legislative proposals, there was evidence of a concern for animals that exceeds that for humans: No cats or dogs, for example, are to be transported in trucks where the van temperature cannot be kept below 85°F.

Does the medical profession really monitor its own performance? One of the essences of a profession is that it assumes certain responsibilities for the competence of its members or the quality of its wares. The importance of this principle was illustrated a decade ago in a dispatch to *The New York Times* from South Africa. As the *Times* reported the meeting, American physicians must have been struck by the similarity to AMA problems:

> Once a year this South African capital, thirty-six miles south of Johannesburg, is the scene of one of the strangest conventions in the world—the meeting of the African Dinga-kaka Association, the organization of South Africa's Witch Doctors. To the most recent meeting this October came 900-odd delegates, some arriving in flashy American-made automobiles, some in jalopies and some on foot. Many of the men wore the conservative gray, brown or black suit one might see on an American country doctor. The women practitioners adorned their native dresses with beads and gaudy feathers. And like convention-goers, all wore delegate badges.
>
> The delegates spent three days listening to discussions of what to do about ten thousand witch doctors practicing outside the four thousand member association; sharing secrets and new discoveries, and watching demonstrations of new techniques.

Like any other professional organization, the Dingakaka has standards which it insists be met. Thus, practitioners who employ such voodoo medicaments as animal bones, skins of snakes and lizards, and potions containing powdered rhinoceros horns and elephant tusks, were denounced as quacks; association members rely primarily on herbs and roots for treatment. Acceptable, however, at the convention apparently were the rolling of bones on the ground as a diagnostic aid and tribal dancing to ward off evil spirits.

One professional attempt to maintain medical standards is in the area of licensing. From their beginning, however, state boards of medical examiners have been handicapped by the fact that they are made up of political appointees of either the party or the medical group in power, rather than experts in the various subjects covered by the examinations. In some states it is specifically required that board members cannot belong to faculties of medical schools. In addition, these boards often have disciplinary and administrative functions that overshadow the duty of giving examinations.

After World War II, the Federation of State Medical Boards of the United States was preoccupied with shortages of physicians and with problems created by graduates of foreign medical schools. In 1956 a permanent committee was appointed with the purpose of creating uniformity in content and quality in state-board examinations. A prime objective became the establishment of universal reciprocity among state boards. The majority of state laws spell out the requirement that endorsement can be offered only to states that have standards equal to their own, and the few states that have interpreted their laws literally and thus avoided a doctrine based on mutual admiration found themselves unable to endorse the licenses of many states. It was found, for example, that nearly half the state boards reported no failures in the examination of 2,000 physicians.

Five years later, the situation was no better. In that year, twenty-six state boards passed every one of the local medical graduates taking the licensure examination, and it is obvious that many of these boards pass all native sons year after year. In 1965, Dr. Robert C. Derbyshire of the federation found that three state boards had not failed a single candidate in ten years, that two states had not failed anyone for nine out of ten years, and four had reported no failures in eight of ten years. The nine states with the lowest failure rate for ten years examined more than 10,000 candidates and refused licensure to only fourteen.

The National Board of Medical Examiners could provide uniformity of standards for the entire country, but some state boards accept the National Board's Diplomates only with reservations, and more than half of the physicians licensed by examination each year prefer to take the state exams. This latter situation is in part related to the lower cost of taking certain state-board examinations, but perhaps even more to their reputation for easiness. In addition, the National Board has expressed no desire to assume legal responsibility for licensure of physicians, feeling that this responsibility must rest with the states. It is content for the moment to try to increase the popularity of its own examinations, which are in general recognized as adequate. It is also willing to provide state boards with tests and questions that may be used by them.

There are strange discrepancies from region to region. One state will require one year of internship of its applicants, whereas others will not. One state may require internship to be of the rotating variety,[3] most do not. Some states require two years of premedical study, others as much as four, and still others require a B.A. or B.S. before the applicant can undertake medical work. Some states will not license a foreign graduate under any circumstances. In 1963, the National Conference of Commissioners on Uniform State Laws drafted a

---

[3] An internship made up of short periods of time spent on a large number of hospital services rather than longer periods on a few services.

model medical-licensure act, but there was not sufficient support to move it further.

There are institutional controls of various kinds. Medical schools are subject to periodic review of their educational programs by national peer groups, and internship and residency training programs are also scrutinized regularly to see that proper training is being afforded. Accredited hospitals must also have "tissue committees" to monitor the quality of surgical competence, and there are often "death-review committees" to review patient fatalities for possible physician culpability. There is little question that such policing actions can affect doctor performance; hospitals have been reported to show a halving in rate of hysterectomies, for example, after the review committees decided that too many normal uteruses were being removed.

The so-called clinical-pathological conferences, where autopsy protocols are reviewed and discussed, can serve as forums for medical reappraisal, but they often are treated as mere detective stories, a game of wit-matching between diagnostician and pathologist, or as opportunity for the exposition of medical oddities and rarities, rather than attempts to see whether a patient might have survived if his medical care had been different. The use of professional consultations and the supervision of house staff are other mechanisms for improving the quality of medical care.

Serious defects remain, however. For example, the medical care that is afforded patients in doctors' offices or on an outpatient basis in hospital clinics is largely unmonitored. The policing is also intrafamilial. Very little of it ever gets to the public's attention. Doctors may lose their right to admit patients to a given hospital, but such physicians usually find it possible to hospitalize their patients at other institutions. Disciplinary reports of the Judicial Council of the AMA annually list only eighty or so revocations of license by state boards, a smaller number of wrist-slappings in the form of "revocations with stay," some forty suspensions, and about forty reprimands or censures. The most frequent reasons for license revocation, however, are not related to medical errors but to abuse of the narcotic license, narcotics addiction, performing illegal abortions, alcoholism, mental incompetency, income-tax evasion, padding of insurance claims, aiding an unlicensed person to practice medicine, and conviction of a crime involving moral turpitude. As the Judicial Council itself pointed out in 1965: ". . . Medicine has not continued its efforts after the discharge of the licensing function. All too seldom are licensed physicians called to task by boards, societies, or colleagues. The Council would hope that greater emphasis be given to ensuring competence and observance of law and ethics after licensure."

The crucial issue in the monitoring of competence among doctors concerns office care. Medical institutions, while far from perfect, exercise a good deal of control over the members of their staff, but some oft-quoted surveys have reported widespread defects in office practice. In the study of general practitioners in North Carolina conducted by Osler L. Peterson, Professor of Preventive Medicine at the Harvard Medical School, 83 per cent of doctors did not usually perform a rectal examination in cases in which the surveying internist thought it was indicated, and two thirds of them gave antibiotics for upper-respiratory infections in a manner that was termed "indiscriminate." Among ninety-three randomly selected general practitioners, history-taking was found to be almost nonexistent. Patients were seldom undressed or asked to lie down for examination, and those with emotional problems were often regarded as hypochondriacs to be disposed of as quickly as possible. *Less than one physician in thirty carried out adequate physical examinations.*[4]

The New York State Society of Internal Medicine requested a group of scientists to devise a methodology for evalu-

---

[4] The chief reason for failure to pass the Boards of Internal Medicine is inability to perform and interpret properly the physical examination.

ating the quality of care being rendered by the society's members in their own offices. A group of physician surveyors checked patient records, looking for the presence or absence of the essential components of a complete record, such as date of first visit, age, sex, history of present illness, past illness, operations, family history, personal, social, and occupational history, physical examination, procedures, recording of diagnosis, treatment, house calls, nursing-home visits, record of hospitalization, etc. Of ninety-one physicians visited, only two thirds kept records that the physician reviewers deemed adequate for nonphysicians to review. (Some of these were merely illegible, but many were incomplete.) They found that being board-certified had little to do with whether the records were adequate or not, but there was a tendency toward decrease in adequacy of records with increase in length of time since graduation from medical school. More adequate records were also kept by those internists who routinely scheduled one hour or more for the patient's first visit, and by those internists with the most laboratory facilities in their offices.

The fact that ten judges, each working independently, showed perfect agreement on the abstracted records shown to them in over half the cases and that in twenty of the twenty-one cases surveyed a clear majority of the judges agreed suggests that there is nothing mysterious about medical practice that makes it impossible for experts to evaluate.

What is badly needed is some way of gauging end results. This is difficult not only because different kinds of patients consult different doctors, so that the challenge presented to physicians is different, but also because there is no clear agreement on the criteria of end results in medicine beyond survival. (Even the latter end point is not unambiguous: a patient may be less interested in survival than in freedom from anxiety or in a patient-doctor relationship that satisfies his particular needs at the moment.)

There is a growing realization that the responsibility of the medical school and university cannot end at its traditional point: the granting of the M.D. degree. Students are for the most part now cut off from the university when they need it most—as they begin to practice medicine. If the universities accept the responsibility for doctor education beyond medical school, where should it end? Logically, with the doctor's death or retirement. The doctor who stops learning rapidly deteriorates; there is no standing still. Unfortunately, postgraduate medical education in America is in a sad state.

Dr. W. Albert Sullivan, Jr., of the University of Minnesota, has lamented that while "great lip service is paid to the subject of continuing the education of the doctor . . . few of the present medical schools consider this as one of their primary responsibilities." Dr. Sullivan pointed out that while sixty-five of the nation's eighty-eight medical schools offer continuation medical courses, a closer scrutiny shows that only 20 per cent or so of schools consider continuation of education important enough to list a department, a division, or a section of postgraduate medical education in the Directory of the Association of American Medical Colleges, and of these schools, only two thirds actually have an active functioning department that regularly and consistently provides instruction for the graduate physician.

Since the same people seem to turn up over and over again at programs conducted for physicians, it would seem that for some reason the medical schools have failed to pique the imagination and interest of the vast majority of practicing doctors. While physicians give reasons such as distance from home town, time away from office, expense, and unavailability of an interesting course, the real problem is probably that the doctor has not been sufficiently motivated to want to learn and that, in Sullivan's words, it is "too comfortable continuing to practice just exactly in the way that he has done for the last 15 years, and thus avoid exposing any intellectual inadequacies which he might have."

Lindsay E. Beaton, vice chairman of the Council on Mental Health of the American Medical Association, has expressed a pessimistic view of both the problem and the hope of solving it:

> These postgraduate schemes assume that a man in the field can be kept professionally spic and span by periodic courses, irregular attendance at meetings, and the rest. They ignore the evident—that only when one lives day by day in the atmosphere of intellectual excitement and scientific transition can he expect to stay young in his learning. The honest truth is that only the doctor in the medical college or the large hospital (usually university-connected) or the major urban clinic, associated with teaching and research as well as with patient care, can truly be considered modern. . . . In medicine, in this land of the free and the taxed, it is the general practitioner, the family physician, the least academic of all men, who needs this fellowship and regular restoration the most.

The medical profession is unwilling to face the serious problem of what to do with the doctor who cannot or will not maintain professional standards but is not actually breaking the law. It seems reasonable that a physician's hospital privileges be related to his competence, and that he be ousted if his performance is inadequate, but some physicians argue that a doctor should not be threatened but in some way convinced that it is his duty to keep up to date and competent. They do not suggest how to do this effectively.

The hospital has a legal responsibility to meet certain minimum standards, and incompetent performance by its physicians should eliminate it from the privilege of accreditation. But an incompetent physician thrown out of one hospital will find another hospital where he is not under comparable supervision. The only solution would seem to be to have state boards revoke such a person's license. It is here that the medical profession balks.

Those who believe that medical societies should require every member to take postgraduate courses and that the profession should find means to evaluate fairly each doctor's practice are motivated by the fear that if medicine does not do this voluntarily, the law will eventually force it to. Commercial airline pilots are subject to regular physical examinations and proficiency tests in order to see whether they remain fit for their job. (A jet pilot who goofs is likely to die as a result of his mistake, along with his victims, but the same is not true for a physician, who lives to see his mistakes buried.) Doctors who are not taking advantage of opportunities to improve their competence are not likely ever to do so without some nonvoluntary regulation.

The American Academy of General Practice insists that each of its 28,000 members submit proof of 150 hours of postgraduate work every three years. Annually some 600 general practitioners are dropped from the academy for failure to do so, although it is not clear what impact this has on their practice—probably none. Specialty societies and AMA member societies do not have similar programs. The American Board of Physical Medicine and the American Board of Urology have in their bylaws statements that a member can lose certification if he refuses to be examined for competence, but neither board is known ever to have invoked the rule. A survey made in 1960 of over a thousand certified specialists show that two thirds favored their boards checking up on them and insisting that they keep up to date.

Because voluntary health insurance pays as much for poor surgery as for good surgery, for bad medicine as for good medicine, there is no economic incentive for maintaining competence. In 1959, Dr. Gunnar Gundersen, then president of the AMA, suggested that the doctor's right to practice should hinge on his taking a recurrent licensure examination, but the AMA promptly disassociated itself from the proposal and the AMA still does not favor compulsory continuing education. Only 25 per cent or so of practicing physicians now take advantage of medical-school courses.

One cannot be encouraged by the possibility that doctors keep themselves abreast of the times by diligent reading of scientific reports. Most doctors receive several medical journals and newspapers, some of which they pay for and a good many of which they receive free. The available information suggests that after doctors read their county medical bulletins (which are mostly related to local matters and not science) they turn to *Medical Economics,* the *Journal of the American Medical Association,* and *Modern Medicine.* The average physician is said to spend forty-five minutes a day reading such material. Caplow, writing in the *Harvard Business Review,* estimated that whereas almost half his sample of physicians read periodicals systematically or regularly, taking notes or at least reading in detail articles and advertisements of special interest, 47 per cent skim the material in an unplanned manner, and 7 per cent do no reading at all.

The pharmaceutical industry has moved with vigor into the void left by inadequate postgraduate medical education. Through throwaway journals, free periodicals subsidized by drug-house advertising, television programs, and exhibits at meetings, the drug houses of America attempt to supply information of all kinds to physicians. They also mail directly to the physician a variety of promotional and informational material, and the industry employs some 15,000 detail men to visit physicians. The detail man serves as a source of information or a reminder to the doctor about the products manufactured by his own firm; but he is basically a salesman and not an educator, although much of the physician's knowledge about pharmaceuticals comes from him.

Although perhaps most physicians attend one or more conventions during the year, when doctors have been polled on this point, about half of them say they go to the meetings to associate with their colleagues, and about a quarter go "to get away for a while." Many hospitals have first-rate teaching sessions, but these conferences are often considered too specialized by the average practicing physician, who seems to find little time to spend at them.

A number of medical schools produce television programs

or radio conferences, including two-way radio conferences between associated hospitals, in an attempt to bring education to
the doctor rather than waiting for the doctor to come to the
source of information. As with other techniques for physician
enlightenment, however, the majority of doctors seem lukewarm about the idea.

In all the concern for maintaining quality of medical
practice, a particular cause of worry is the general practitioner,
who poses problems both different and more serious than those
of the specialist. Late in 1963, the World Health Organization
announced that the general practitioner had reached a cross-
roads in the more highly developed countries, and that the
future might witness his extinction. In 1931, the United States
listed 112,000 general practitioners and 22,000 full-time specialists. By 1965 only 69,000 of the quarter million or so doctors
who had completed their formal training classified themselves
as general practitioners, and in recent estimates only 20 per
cent of medical-school graduates seem headed for general
practice.

One reason for the change is the great increase in the accumulated knowledge that now constitutes the hard core of
scientific medicine. Fifty years ago it was still possible for a
conscientious physician to master what had to be known about
medical ills. Today the majority of medical-school graduates
select one segment of modern medicine rather than attempt to
play Renaissance man. Our medical schools not only reflect this
trend, they accelerate it. The student quickly observes that the
most distinguished faculty members are specialists and are
awarded not only fame and prestige, but also the most exciting
diagnostic and therapeutic problems. Not lost upon him,
either, is a certain professorial condescension toward the lowly
GP. It is not surprising that one third of the students aiming
for general practice when they enter medical school have given
up the idea by graduation.

A second powerful force affecting the general practitioner
has been urbanization. In a community only large enough to

support one doctor, the doctor must tackle as best he can whatever medical problems arise. But a population that increasingly
congregates in cities or in suburbs of large cities, where specialists abound, is less apt to rely on the Jack-of-all-trades who is
master of none. To some, in and out of the medical profession,
the general practitioner in today's urban society is a flagrant
anachronism, and modern medicine is that practiced by specialists working singly or in group practice.

Notwithstanding the apparent reasonableness of these
arguments, the fact is that the GP has not disappeared. Thousands of such physicians continue to practice medicine to their
own satisfaction and to that of their patients. In 1947 these
practictioners formed the American Academy of General Practice, second in size only to the American Medical Association.
The AMA has established a Section on General Practice and a
category of residence training in general practice, and each year
grants an award to the General Practitioner of the Year. In
Canada the trend to specialization has leveled off since 1959,
and at present half the graduates there head for general practice. In tradition-laden Scotland, the University of Edinburgh
created the first chair of Medicine in Relation to General
Practice a few years ago. But one wonders if these are merely
delaying tactics, attempts to roll back an inevitable tide of
specialization, or if there is good reason for the refusal of the
GP to lie down and play dead.

Today's generalist is not the romantic horse-and-buggy
doctor of old, traveling long distances in sunshine or storm,
at early morn or midnight, to help usher in the breath of life
or ease the pain and sorrow of death. Except in isolated rural
areas, the office is the main base of activities. Practitioners do
not spend most of their time racing to homes[5] to deliver babies
or set bones. They rarely perform appendectomies in hospital
operating rooms, let alone on kitchen tables. (A cynical GP,

[5] GP's, like specialists, have mostly given up the practice of making house
calls, a decision that may be scientifically defensible but has antagonized many
patients.

refused operating privileges in his local hospital, once wryly observed that a kitchen table was about the only place he could perform an appendectomy.) What the generalist does practice is a family medicine that combines obstetrics, pediatrics, internal medicine, psychiatry, and minor office surgery.

The generalist may work alone or with one or more colleagues; the latter arrangement helps provide coverage at night, on weekends, and during vacations. He is often aided considerably by a nurse assistant and by a technician who attends to such things as blood counts and urinalyses. (Complicated diagnostic tests are handled by outside laboratories and specialists.) An average day will see twenty-five patients coming to the office, the majority with appointments at closely set intervals, but some showing up unexpectedly. Most of the problems are handled without outside help, but perplexing cases call for specialist consultation, which under ideal conditions is asked for and given in an atmosphere of cooperation and mutual respect.

For at least part of the community, such a generalist fills an important need, in spite of specialization, urbanization, and strong antigeneralist trends within the universities and the profession itself. Nor should such preferences be glibly ascribed to the fact that laymen are too ignorant to know bad care when they get it. One consideration is that doctors are chosen as much for their extra-scientific qualities as for their medical qualifications. A charming bedside manner may mask an intellectual or ethical vacuum, but the practice of medicine does involve more than the application of technical know-how and scientific rigor. The physician is not merely a craftsman repairing a complicated piece of machinery; sick people are not depersonalized because they are ill. Most patients do not wish, in the words of Prof. Milton Roemer, to be "cured of a once-fatal disease by someone whose name [they] didn't quite catch."

The physician is best equipped to treat illness when he truly knows his patient—not merely his disturbed physiology, but his emotional history, his habits, his foibles. Lifelong routines cannot be lightly altered, even to treat disease. The choice of remedies, of diagnostic measures, of how much to tell the patient is all conditioned by the nature of the rapport between doctor and patient. Success in these interpersonal relationships does not belong any more naturally to the specialist than to the generalist. It is a matter of humanity, not training, and if a GP possesses it, there is good reason for the consumer to seek him out.[6]

Hippocrates said, twenty-four centuries ago: "For where there is love of man, there is also love of the art. For some patients, though conscious that their position is perilous, recover their health simply through their contentment with . . . the physician." Advances in medical science have, to be sure, increased the number of situations where it is not sufficient to have a physician who is primarily a friend and adviser. The man whose life is threatened by a complicated infection, or the child whose cardiac anomaly requires surgical correction, demands technical expertness—from a misanthrope, if need be. But there still remains an enormous range of human illness, from neurosis to disseminated cancer, where "magic bullets" are lacking and where personal considerations override manual skill or special training.

There is another important attraction for some patients in the concept of continuity of care. Having the same family doctor for years has an ancient and justifiable appeal. One of George Eliot's characters remarked: "It's no trifle at her time of life to part with a doctor who knows her constitution." It can be argued that long-term care could be provided as well by a specialist. But there is particular meaning for many in a doctor who can handle a baby's birth, his childhood diseases, and the problems of adulthood, and who furthermore cares for all members of the family at the same time. At least theoretically,

---

[6] It should be pointed out, however, that a poll of patients in 1962 showed specialists rated higher than GP's on such items as "taking interest in his patients" and "treating each patient as a human being."

this opportunity to know the problems and personalities of an entire family permits a more comprehensive and informed type of medical service. Indeed, certain internists conduct their practice along just such lines.

A third factor is the matter of costs. The bill for a given illness may vary considerably from doctor to doctor. The fees are not invariably (or even usually) higher if care is given by a specialist, but in some situations this turns out to be the case. Many healthy young women could be delivered safely by a midwife, and a low-income family may find it difficult to justify the services of a specialist for every pregnancy, if the specialist's fee is substantially higher. The process of delivery in more than 90 per cent of cases has been compared to signaling for a fair catch, and if this offends the sensibilities of some, it is nonetheless remarkably close to the truth.

It is expensive to use a different physician for each complaint. A narrowly specialized physician who sends a woman to a dermatologist for her acne, a gynecologist for her routine pelvic checkup, and a psychiatrist for her minor anxieties is certain to increase the cost of medical care for his "patient," who may justifiably come to think of him as a travel agent rather than a doctor. He is also likely to be dropped by the patient; few people like to be treated by committee. As Martial said in the first century A.D.: "Cascellius extracts an aching tooth. Hyginus burns away the hairs that hurt the eyes . . . Hermes is a very Podalirius in curing hernia; but tell me, Gallus, where is he that can help my harassed person?"

One may still ask, however, whether such fragmented medical care is better, medically, than the more convenient and less expensive Jack-of-all-trades approach. If costs were not a problem, should one see specialists for most ailments? After all, one does go to a dentist for a toothache, not to the GP. There is no easy answer. It depends on what the patient is like, what his doctor is like, and what the trouble is.

The owner of a specialty-board diploma is by no means

automatically superior to the doctor who doesn't have one, although he is likely to have stood higher in his graduating class than the nonspecialist. The specialty boards have unquestionably raised the quality of medical care, but they have also been attacked as restrictive, monopolistic, arrogant, and less concerned with true ability than with rigid requirements. It is, furthermore, important not only how well trained a man has been, but how well he maintains his medical knowledge. There are specialists who fail to keep their critical faculties sharply honed over the years, and there are conscientious GP's who do keep abreast of medical progress and practice medicine superbly.

There is, then, a case to be made for the family doctor. The WHO Expert Committee on General Practice has asserted that the GP is "an irreplaceable element in the fight against disease." Other groups in many countries have called for a renascence of the family doctor and the "first-line" physician, urging society to find some means of keeping and improving its GP's.

One pressing need is for long-range economic aid. At present, the decision to enter general practice right after internship (which is undesirable almost 100 per cent of the time) is at times dictated less by intellectual sloth than by unwillingness to incur further debt. Society is thus faced with the paradox of the least formal training being given the man who needs the most—the practitioner who will have to treat the broadest possible spectrum of human ills.

Programs to train the generalist require expansion and revision, plus provisions for continuing exposure over the years to the finest possible teaching. A few countries, such as Israel and Yugoslavia, are experimenting with new schemes that may suggest improvements for our own programs. The program at Zagreb is perhaps the most impressive vocational training for general practitioners available anywhere in the world. Since 1960, doctors who have been in practice for a minimal period can take a three-year course, which runs a full afternoon every week, plus three periods when the doctor is provided with a replacement and goes back for hospital training. Since this program began, Yugoslav GP's have experienced a transfusion of self-confidence, are more readily accepted as equals by specialists, and are more often sought out by patients. They also get paid more than doctors who have not taken the course.

The Academy of General Practice, much distressed over the decline and fall of the GP, has mounted a major campaign to make a specialist out of the family doctor. It has suggested a three-year postgraduate course, with emphasis on such subjects as preventive medicine, psychology, sociology, and anthropology, and board certification. Dr. Amos N. Johnson, former president of the academy, has estimated that such training would suit the GP to provide for 80 per cent of the medical needs of society, including preventive medicine as well as remedial care. The AMA House of Delegates has backed the move and authorized the necessary planning by its Council on Medical Education. (Many GP's who originally joined the Academy of General Practice to avoid board-certification problems now find themselves with no place to hide.)

All the discussions about bringing together specialists, teachers, and the man in practice may come to naught, however, if the town-gown syndrome is not cured. Within the profession hard feelings exist on many fronts. Some doctors do not refer patients to a university hospital because they allegedly never get a follow-up from the medical center and never see the patients again. Other physicians bridle at the publicity accorded researchers at the medical institutions, with the implication that only there are first-class medical services available. Medical societies frequently resent medical-school expansion and full-time salaried service, as well as competition for patients between society members and medical-school staff. Medical-school faculty members are accused of living off the taxpayers and of not earning an honest living.

The academician is criticized for his ivory-tower attitude and his emphasis on rare diseases, for being more interested in book learning than in actual clinical experience, and for focusing on laboratory tests rather than clinical skills. Slates of town-versus-gown candidates for medical-society offices are frequently put up, with bitter political contests and elections. The medical school is often considered a monolith by the downtown practitioners, who think of themselves as individuals opposing a massive enemy. The result of all this is to damage the prestige of institutions and tarnish the reputations of individuals and the medical profession.

The most comprehensive study of the town-gown fight has been conducted by Patricia L. Kendall of the Bureau of Applied Social Research at Columbia University. Personal interviews were held in eight communities in which there was a medical school. Both the medical educators and the medical practitioners in these communities agreed that there was a growing emphasis on research in medical schools. The medical educators tended to look on this favorably, the practicing physicians unfavorably. It was also agreed that there is a trend in most medical schools to replace part-time teachers with full-time staff; most medical educators favored this development, but many practitioners viewed it with alarm. The medical educators approve the fact that a patient in a university hospital is often seen by many consultants, whereas practitioners find such a system of consultations irritating and annoying. The fact that physicians of high caliber fill the staffs of medical schools is viewed with pride by faculty members, but is considered a threat by some practitioners. There is a discontent engendered by the fact that many postgraduate courses have a high scientific content. The medical educators state that this is because they do not wish to create a double standard for practitioners and specialists; the general practitioners, on the other hand, are frustrated, since they would prefer to obtain "practical advice" for treating patients, rather than theoretical concepts.

Private practice by full-time faculty members is a source of obvious discontent. In favor of such practice is the fact that the medical school has certain needs in regard to training and teaching, that these can only be served by such patient care, and that high-level private practice contributes to the welfare of the community. Those who argue against academic private practice claim that it interferes with the teaching responsibilities of faculty members, and also that it competes economically with local practitioners. But while practitioners fear that they may lose patients to salaried hospital doctors, this seems to occur only rarely. Most doctors in the communities studied seem to have as much work as they want and would find it difficult to assume responsibility for any more patients.

The public, often unaware of these struggles and animosities, is caught in the cross fire. Most doctors are not gowners but towners, and it is they who provide the public with the bulk of everyday health care. But it is the academicians who train the embryonic doctor when he is a medical student, it is they who are at the forefront of medical progress, and it is they who control the big teaching hospitals that provide the medical skills and the opportunity for continuing education doctors so urgently require. What good will it do to develop grand schemes for bridging the intellectual gap between town and gown if there is a growing emotional gap too broad to be spanned? The public does not benefit from fruitless bickering between these segments of the health professions. It is too early to tell if society will solve the problem of maintaining a high competence in its medical practitioners, but it is certain to fail if the building blocks in any proposed structure for monitoring and upgrading the quality of medical care cannot be mortised together.

4

An Ounce
of Prevention

I N THE PROVOCATIVE and occasionally outrageous preface to
The Doctor's Dilemma, Bernard Shaw makes the following observation: "Until the medical profession becomes a body
of men trained and paid by the country to keep the country in
health it will remain what it is at present: a conspiracy to
exploit popular credulity and suffering." This was written in
1911, but more than half a century later its call for more
emphasis on the prophylaxis of illness and less preoccupation
with remedial action is still appropriate.

There is no question but that it is better to prevent disease than to have to treat it, especially since many of our most
dreaded medical killers are not amenable to cure. But preventive medicine in its broad sense is more than the prevention
of disease. It includes the promotion of health and the prevention of increasing disability by rehabilitating those already
damaged by disease.

The effective range of preventive medicine can be illustrated by considering a time-honored public problem such as
syphilis. At the level of health promotion, health education and
hygiene, sex education, and preparation for marriage can be
taught. Society can arrange premarital examinations, attend to

personality development, and generally improve socioeconomic conditions and recreational facilities. At the level of specific protection, chemical, mechanical, or chemotherapeutic prophylaxis can be used, the avoidance of sexual promiscuity urged, prenatal blood tests performed, and social action taken against commercialized prostitution. The next level is that of early diagnosis and therapy, which involves case finding, investigation of contacts, examination of infants born of syphilitic mothers, as well as prompt treatment to destroy the disease-producing organisms. At the level of limiting disability, there is case finding of latent or late syphilis and low-cost facilities for treating complications of syphilis. In terms of rehabilitation, one must think of both the medical and the social problems of those rendered blind, or cardiologically or psychiatrically disabled, by syphilis.

Hugh R. Leavell and E. Gurney Clark have nicely pointed out the difference between the preventive medical practices of the public health expert and the private doctor. The public-health expert is trained as a specialist in preventive medicine, which is what primarily concerns him. His "patient" is the community—groups rather than individuals—and it is the community to which he is responsible. He is more than willing to accept failure of a health procedure for a few if the majority benefits from the procedure. He is attuned to the need for persuading people to avail themselves of medical services, has legal backing in some of his community efforts, and is financed largely by tax funds.

In contrast, the individual practitioner of medicine is not a specialist in preventive medicine and indeed is usually ill prepared for this role. His whole background is attuned to treatment, not prevention. His patient is the individual, not the group, and it is the individual to whom he is responsible. He is in general aiming at successful treatment of each patient and does not consider failure with a few patients compensated for by success with many. He is bound by medical ethics not to advertise his services, has no legal authority beyond the right to practice, and is usually paid by individual fees, with or without insurance coverage.

For a variety of reasons, the prevention of disease has in many respects drifted from the hands of the individual doctors into community health services. Such problems as water purification or pasteurization of milk are obviously not suited to individual action, but the health department has even invaded the doctor's territory in regard to preventive measures that require individual treatment, such as in cases of tuberculosis or venereal disease. The trend has been encouraged by failure to educate the public to pay for preventive services other than those supplied by pediatricians, obstetricians, and dentists. For other services that a practitioner might provide in promoting health, there are no efficient methods of payment. The increase in specialization and the decline of the family doctor have also influenced the public to search for doctors to deal with specific symptoms, not anything as vague as "health" or "hygiene." Finally, doctors themselves are more likely to be attracted to the drama of therapy than to the blandness of preventive measures.

This chapter will focus on a few highly important and preventable medical ailments that are or should be of considerable interest to physicians either because research is needed on the problems or because doctors need to serve as lobbyists attempting to change society. I hope to reinforce the proposition that doctors have great contributions to make to society in this area, were they but willing to shoulder the task more fully.

I will begin with a problem that is ordinarily not considered within the realm of preventive medicine—vehicular traffic accidents. Everyone would agree on the magnitude of the problem. The trend is continually upward, year by year, and at present the annual U.S. death toll is equivalent to what would result from the annual sinking of twenty giant ocean liners with all hands on board, or ten jet airplane crashes per week. There are more than 50,000 deaths and 4,000,000 injuries each year; automobiles are responsible for more deaths than anything else except cancer and cardiovascular disease. For young people between the ages of fifteen and twenty-four, the automobile is the first cause of death, and one out of every two Americans can expect to be in an injury-producing collision during his lifetime. If the number of automobiles continues to increase at the present rate, the annual death rate from the automobile should be more than 100,000 in the next decade, with the cost of accidents climbing to $15,000,000,000 per year.

Physicians have good cause to be concerned about automobile accidents. Not only are they, like other citizens, likely to be personally involved in such catastrophes, but it is they who are responsible for providing medical and surgical care to accident victims. The most severely injured will require intensive emergency and rehabilitative treatment. Neurosurgeons, orthopedic surgeons, and plastic surgeons frequently are called upon to apply their skills. Doctors also have special reason to be aware of the medical disabilities that contribute to accidents, and of the possibility that alcohol and various drugs may induce automobile fatalities and injuries.

Dr. William Haddon, Jr., first director of the new National Traffic Safety Agency, has declared:

> It is about time that members of the medical profession, who regard this as an exotic and nonmedical area, begin to understand its place in their traditional concerns. Unless they do so and begin to address themselves to its problems, there will continue to be no professional group centrally related to this field. . . . the physicians now graduating are fantastically ill informed as far as this field is concerned.

Dr. Haddon believes doctors should start by first ensuring that emergency services in their areas are modern and efficient. Such services do not, in most parts of the country, come within the professional concern of physicians, although it is hard to see who else should take on this job. While efficient methods have been developed for retrieving and treating the wounded in wartime, these are not applied on the domestic scene.

Another concern of Dr. Haddon is with the paucity of research on the basic mechanisms of injury in vehicular accidents:

> If someone had done a proper job in 1910 of finding out what it was that was killing people, that is, that structures such as the steering shaft were coming through the drivers' chests, we might have long ago achieved the better packaging that is now beginning to become evident in the newer vehicles.

Not all physicians have avoided these problems. For example, E. S. Gurdjian and his colleagues at Wayne State University have performed a series of fascinating experiments with cadaver heads, seeking to obtain basic information on the role of crash forces in producing trauma. It has been reported that 70 to 80 per cent of all deaths and injuries in crash decelerations are from face or head injuries caused by the body or the head striking surrounding structures with less give than the head.

A variety of studies at Wayne, Cornell, and the Federal Aviation Agency Laboratory at Oklahoma City have shed light on the needless loss of life and facial destruction in crash impacts. In most vehicles, people are surrounded by rigid tubes, knobs, door posts, and sharp instruments—all beautifully calculated to maim the face and head. The available data indicate that if this environment were changed to a medium-weight deformable metal, without a heavy structure directly behind it, the impact load would be distributed over the area of the face and it would be almost impossible to produce facial and forehead fractures in crashes. Damage to the brain would then be feared primarily from forces capable of producing brain lacerations without intermediary skull fracture.

If an automobile passenger is not wearing a seatbelt, rapid deceleration will propel him through the windshield. But as a larger number of people start wearing seatbelts, the potential hazard of the dash panel will increase. The padded lip available in cars of more recent vintage may actually make the dashboard more dangerous, since the face usually comes in contact with the heavy structure that has been added to attach the padded lip.

What is especially depressing about Detroit's apathy in initiating change is the fact that knowledgeable scientists have long known about auto deficiencies. The need to revise the instrument panels in automobiles, for example, was pointed out by farsighted physicians years ago. In the 1930's, the late Dr. Claire Straith, a plastic surgeon from Detroit, begged the car industry to provide panels to protect the crashing motorist. In 1948, Dr. Fletcher Woodward pointed out to the automobile industry the design features of automobiles that were producing death and injuries, and was promptly labeled a crackpot by one car producer. The same producer berated the American College of Surgeons for formally suggesting needed design features to the automobile manufacturers.

When Dr. Haddon was made director of the National Traffic Safety Agency and new standards of auto-safety design were promulgated by the government, there were high hopes for a quick resolution to the safety problems facing the public. It was expected that the 1968 vehicles would be a great improvement over previous years. Unfortunately, various circumstances seem to have resulted in a watering down of the original demands on the automobile industry. Dr. Haddon believes that significant progress has been made, and that companies must be given sufficient time to adjust to the new legislation. Other physicians, less kindly in their attitudes, have described the regulations as everything from compromise to surrender, and some have called for a new congressional inquiry. It is perhaps not surprising that an industry that has dragged its wheels for several decades is unable to move rapidly enough in one year to achieve desired goals.

Physicians could make their impact felt in still other ways. It has, for example, been shown that physician involvement in planning educational efforts to convince consumers of the importance of equipping automobiles with seatbelts can pay off. In Pittsburgh and in Indiana substantial gains have been made by efficiently planned promotion efforts, in Pittsburgh conducted personally by a practicing pediatrician in face-to-face discussions with parents of his patients, in Indiana by a committee working under the auspices of the Public Health Service, the American Medical Association, and the National Safety Council. Similar efforts by other medical groups and individuals, utilizing the privileged position and prestige of the doctor, could provide substantial benefits to society.

Another opportunity for interaction between doctors and the public in regard to traffic safety relates to the clear evidence that alcohol contributes significantly to auto accidents. In pioneering investigations conducted under the leadership of Dr. Haddon before he entered federal service, it was found that blood alcohol concentrations drawn routinely from people killed in traffic accidents showed that 70 per cent of those tested were legally intoxicated. About 30 per cent of pedestrians killed by cars showed such alcohol concentrations.

From other studies, it would appear that a majority of drivers and pedestrians involved in traffic accidents after drinking are not social drinkers but inebriates, with the possible exception of younger drivers. Indeed, most fatally injured pedestrians seem to be afflicted either by extreme youth, old age, or intoxication, and there is need to pay special attention to these factors if such fatalities are to be diminished.

In contrast to the situation in some countries, such as Sweden, the American alcoholic driver is often not effectively restricted from driving or required to seek treatment. Means have to be found to detect and treat the chronically alcoholic driver when he is brought in for minor traffic violations. The traditional patient-doctor relationship prevents the physician from supplying information that might help to achieve these goals. Perhaps what is needed for such violators are alcoholic clinics, which can operate in a medical rather than a legal atmosphere. This is an example of the conflict between the physician's responsibility to the individual and his responsibility to society. If a doctor refuses to help society prevent a chronic alcoholic patient from driving, he is protecting his patient from inconvenience, but at the risk of serious damage to the patient himself and to the rest of the population. Yet both ethical and legal restrictions impede the physician with a sense of social responsibility in this matter.

Another scientific pioneer in highway-safety study is Ross A. McFarland, of the Harvard School of Public Health. He has been interested in the attitudes and personal characteristics of drivers repeatedly involved in accidents. The personality structure of the accident repeater has been described as eccentric, impulsive, or mildly psychopathic. In comparing truck drivers who are accident-free with the accident repeaters, McFarland and his colleagues found that the accident repeaters were more likely to show minor violations in their motor vehicle records, court records of offenses against persons and property, and unfavorable business inspection reports.

Fatigue is a predisposing factor. Subjects do less well on a variety of psychological and psychomotor tasks after prolonged driving. Driving performance deteriorates in characteristic ways. Fatigue initially affects the timing of reactions. In later stages, gross mistakes appear, but at first it is more likely that the right response is made at the wrong time. As fatigue increases, certain stimuli are ignored and important responses are omitted. The operator thinks he is doing as well as previously, but he is actually operating less skillfully and may miscalculate the seriousness of a situation. Under conditions of extreme fatigue, drivers may experience hallucinations and have accidents by maneuvering to avoid collision with imaginary obstacles. This seems most likely to occur on long-distance runs at night, when there is little to stimulate the driver and he feels sleepy.

ONE OF THE AREAS of preventive medicine that has been accorded a great deal of discussion in recent years is the study of the host of illnesses associated with cigarette smoking. Criticism of smoking is not new to our own times. Early critics included King James I of England and Robert Burton, who attacked "hellish, devilish and damned tobacco" in *The Anatomy of Melancholy*. In the nineteenth century some French physicians related smoking to both angina pectoris and cancer of the oral cavity, and in the late 1930's investigators in several countries began to produce cancer in rabbits and mice with extracts of tobacco smoke. Shortly thereafter, the American surgeons Alton Ochsner and Michael De Bakey were struck by the fact that every one of their patients with lung cancer, with the exception of two women, had been an excessive smoker.

Since that time, an impressive group of prospective and retrospective studies have tackled the relationship between smoking and disease. They have all come to similar conclusions.

Men who have never smoked seem to have the lowest death rate, occasional smokers are a trifle higher, cigar and pipe smokers a bit higher, but not much. Indeed, pipe smokers and nonsmokers have almost the same death rates except for cancer of the mouth, larynx, and lip. The highest rates are shown by those men who smoke cigarettes, and the more you smoke the greater is the probability of dying. The degree of inhalation is also directly related to the risk. Ex-smokers who have stopped for several years—it is necessary to observe this time period to allow elimination from the figures of people who have stopped smoking because they were so seriously ill—have lower death rates than those who continue. Accidents, violent deaths, and suicide are not related to smoking habits, but all other broad categories of cause of death are, including heart and circulatory disease, cancer, pulmonary disease other than cancer, and all other diseases. There is a higher death rate from lung cancer in cities than in rural areas for both smokers and nonsmokers, but the urban-rural difference is trivial compared with the difference between smokers and nonsmokers.

Women also face hazards from smoking, although smoking remains more dangerous for men than for women. Thus for males the lung-cancer death rate among smokers is 111 deaths per 100,000 per year, as against 12 per 100,000 in nonsmokers. For women, the figures are 35 and 7. A possible explanation is that women are less exposed to cigarette smoke than male smokers of the same ages, as judged by the number of cigarettes smoked per day, the degree of inhalation, and the number of years they have indulged in the habit. In addition, regardless of smoking habits, men usually have higher death rates from most diseases.

The notion that cigarette smoking and respiratory disease are related is highly strengthened by an analysis of 11,000 Seventh-Day Adventist men living in California. This group is similar to other men except for occupation, an older age distribution, and much less tobacco exposure. The total number of deaths observed and the deaths from respiratory disease were approximately one half and one fourth, respectively, that expected at comparable ages for California men. In the Seventh-Day Adventist group, the twenty-eight deaths contributed to by emphysema or lung cancer were concentrated in a minority with a history of heavy tobacco usage. Only one such death occurred among the 35 per cent of lifetime Seventh-Day Adventists who had never smoked.

While some have attacked the correlation between smoking and all kinds of diseases as tending to weaken the argument that cause and effect are involved, investigation of some of the weirder relationships has adduced evidence that may help explain the phenomenon. Bladder cancer, for example, has long been known to be capable of being induced by certain chemicals, such as naphthylamine. Workers engaged in the hazardous production of related chemicals are now protected as a consequence of this knowledge, but the incidence of bladder carcinoma in the general population is rising. Evidence from Canada shows that urinary excretion of carcinogenic metabolites of the normal amino acid tryptophan, similar to the carcinogens that cause industrial bladder cancer, rises considerably during smoking, and suggests that smoking may contribute to bladder cancer by inhibiting the normal metabolism of tryptophan.

A similar consideration applies to the increased incidence of coronary-artery disease among smokers. In various surveys, there has been a clear-cut relationship between the magnitude of cigarette smoking and both the presence of atherosclerosis in the coronary arteries and the incidence of heart attacks and sudden death. While it is not clear how this works in a cause-and-effect sense, some interesting studies during the past few years make the association possibly less mysterious. It has, for example, been reported that in habitual smokers the clotting time of the blood is decreased soon after cigarette smoking. In addition, dogs given daily injections of nicotine for a six-week period showed a 50 per cent increase in the average cholesterol concentration in their serum, an elevation that was maintained until the administration of nicotine stopped. Dogs have even been given cigarettes to "smoke," by a technique that involves placing a cigarette over the intake valve of a respirator and then breathing for the animals through a hole in the trachea. Such animals have shown dramatic changes in heart rate and rhythm, and large increases in blood pressure. Human beings given a cigarette to smoke or an injection of nicotine also demonstrate significant abnormalities in the ballistocardiogram, a means of measuring the contractile force of the heart as well as the resilience of the circulatory system.

Emphysema is a deadly disease, for which there has been an increase in annual deaths in the United States from 3,000 in 1953 to 17,600 in 1963. Emphysema is thirteen times more prevalent among cigarette smokers than among nonsmokers, and it is estimated that from 1,000,000 to 10,000,000 Americans are afflicted to some extent by the diease. It is more widespread than lung cancer and tuberculosis combined, and almost as prevalent as arthritis. The disease is characterized by degenerative changes in the walls of the tiny air sacs in the lungs in which there is an exchange of oxygen and carbon dioxide during respiration. How cigarette smoking may exert its deleterious effects is not known, but there are a number of reasonable theories. The irritating nature of cigarette smoke can produce inflammation of the air passages and other lung structures. With damage to these structures, there ensues a chain of events including chronic cough, infection, and a variety of pathological changes due to recurrent cycles of inflammation and infection, plus the mechanical stresses imposed by repeated coughing. Dogs subjected to daily cigarette smoking via the method described above have shown a rise in the viscosity of the blood, a marked increase in heart weight relative to body weight, and pulmonary fibrosis and emphysema similar to the human disease states. Studies at the University of California on pulmonary function in smokers and nonsmokers have shown various changes, with a deleterious effect on ventilatory function from cigarette smoking approximately equivalent to two decades of aging. Furthermore, autopsy studies on the bronchial tree and the air sacs show all sorts of changes in smokers, ranging from emphysema and fibrosis to premalignant changes.

One of the most frightening aspects of the relationship between cigarette smoking and health is the problem of lung cancer. The World Health Organization in 1965 issued statistics showing that the mortality rate from this disease has doubled in the last ten years. An alarming increase in such deaths has been recorded in both Europe and North America. In addition to the direct irritating effects of smoke already described, some Harvard investigators have studied the possible contribution of a radioactive element named polonium[210], a naturally occurring daughter-isotope of radium, trace amounts of which are present in cigarette smoke. Polonium[210] was found in higher concentrations in the lung tissue of individuals smoking cigarettes than in the lungs of nonsmokers. These investigators estimated that the cumulative local dose of radiation to certain small regions of bronchial tissue where the polonium is concentrated may be quite high and that this radioactive ingredient may be an important factor in the initiation of bronchial carcinoma in man.

Regrettably, warnings about tobacco have never had much lasting effect on the populace. Charles I placed a heavy tax on tobacco, which proved a great source of revenue but not a psychological restraint, the English being clearly unimpressed by the king's arguments and his appeals to their good sense. Pope Urban VIII, who issued a decree of excommunication against those who took snuff in church, and Pope Innocent XII, who issued a similar decree at the turn of the eighteenth century against smoking, were apparently equally unsuccessful. The authorities at Berne in 1661 inscribed their prohibition against smoking on the church tablet containing the Ten Commandments, immediately under the Commandment "Thou shalt not commit adultery," but there is no evidence that this technique was any more effective.

Despite *Smoking and Health,* the widely publicized Public Health Service report condemning tobacco as a health hazard, remarkably little has happened to cigarette smoking in this country. Even with a warning label on every package of cigarettes since January 1966, U.S. Department of Agriculture figures for domestic consumption for 1966 showed a record 525,000,000,000 cigarettes, up nearly 3 per cent over the year before. The biggest change has been a shift to filter cigarettes, despite the lack of evidence that all such filters help screen out tar and nicotine. (Some filter cigarettes actually seem to let through more tar and nicotine than do many unfiltered cigarettes.) In addition, a certain number of adult smokers have given up smoking for ill health or other reasons, and the curve of increase is a little less steep than one would have anticipated on the basis of projected past trends.

Why has there been so little impact on the smoking habits of the nation? To begin with, there is continued propaganda from the tobacco industry questioning the relationship between cigarette smoking and disease. As the Australian pharmacologist Adrien Albert once said: "Most of the tobacco industry seems to be of the opinion that cigarette smoking is not of itself dangerous and that the real trouble is some extraneous factor which they hope to eliminate. To me, this sounds faintly as though the Hoist and Scaffolding Manufacturers' Association has found that falling from a high building is not of itself dangerous, and that there must be an extraneous factor such as, for instance, hitting the ground." The industry has also propagandized on behalf of the notion of self-regulation, and has expressed itself in favor of altering advertising to eliminate allusions to the notion that smoking is "essential to social prominence, distinction, success, or sexual attraction," and of not distributing sample cigarettes to persons under twenty-one years of age.

There are also economic and political overtones. Tobacco is the fifth-largest cash crop in the country, and provides many millions of dollars in wages for thousands of employees. A great deal of money goes to the federal, state, and local governments in excise taxes, and the tobacco industry is a prime advertiser in many communications media.

In addition, part of the explanation lies in the psychology of the cigarette smoker. After the initial flurry of excitement over the Surgeon General's report, there was a significant drop in cigarette sales, but this trend quickly reversed itself. A study by Dr. James W. Swinehart of the University of Michigan School of Public Health has shed some light on the reaction of people to the report. A questionnaire was given to 128 university students two weeks after the report was published. They were asked such things as whether they accepted the findings of the report, whether they believed that they were susceptible to the diseases said to threaten smokers, and whether they planned to change their smoking behavior. Similar questionnaires were given two weeks, and again two and a half months, later. During the period of study there was an increase of smoking and a decrease in acceptance of the report, recall of its findings, and endorsement of governmental actions with regard to smoking and health. Dr. Swinehart concluded that messages repeated too often become ineffective and that threatening messages about the harm that can come from smoking eventually incur hostility toward the person who keeps urging the subject. His second conclusion is that harping on negative factors such as the bodily damage that may result from smoking is not very effective, since people can always justify what they want to do or what they are trapped into doing by habit.

There is also the difficulty that comes from a deleterious effect that appears only a long time after exposure. If people were to experience chest pain, spit blood, or have respiratory distress every time they smoked a cigarette, they would be less likely to acquire the habit. Even dramatic physical distress is not likely to have much effect once the habit is thoroughly ingrained, however. Doctors have all seen patients gasping for breath from emphysema who agree in theory that smoking is bad for their lungs, but who nevertheless can always be found with a cigarette dangling from their lips.

Cigarette smoking in many heavy smokers, if not most, is probably a form of true addiction. Heavier smokers have been observed in the state of sudden abstinence from smoking, and contrasted with a comparable group of subjects allowed to smoke whenever they wished. There were symptoms of distress, as well as changes in heart rate and blood pressure. These findings occurred even when low-nicotine cigarettes were substituted for high-nicotine cigarettes. The words used by smokers and their compulsive searching out of cigarettes while attempting to break the habit are reminiscent of the behavior of narcotics addicts and alcoholics.

Because of all these facts, and because nearly half the high-school seniors who have reached the age of eighteen years have already begun to smoke cigarettes with some degree of regularity, it appears important to prevent the habit rather than try to cure it. There are some data that explain why teenagers smoke. To begin with, it is very important if the parents smoke. If both do, then a third of the children smoke. If only one parent smokes, this figure drops to 25 per cent, and it is 15 per cent if neither parent smokes. A second driving force is the failure to achieve status among one's peers or to achieve other satisfactions. Smoking is high among those who have fallen behind their peers in school, those who do not participate in extracurricular activities, and those who are taking the scholastically less demanding courses in school. One study of a large sample of college freshmen indicated a clear correlation between freshman grades and smoking habits: the higher the grades, the lower the percentage of smokers. With at least some youngsters, one motivation is rebellion, a defiance of parental prohibitions.

The campaign against cigarette smoking has been marred by indications that the medical profession is itself in disagreement about the harm that tobacco can cause. Some individual physicians have been outspoken in their denunciation of smoking; so have such voluntary foundations as the American Cancer Society and the National Tuberculosis Association. Other doctors have denied that any convincing evidence exists. The American Medical Association confused the matter magnificently by simultaneously taking an agnostic stand on the Surgeon General's report and $5,000,000 from the tobacco industry to research the problem. A public already all too inclined to smoke is not likely to be swayed by reports that suggest massive uncertainty within the ranks of medicine.

Surveys indicate that physicians who are either nonsmokers or ex-smokers outnumber tobacco users by two to one. Of 1,440 doctors participating in a poll conducted by *Medical Tribune*, 27 per cent said that they had never smoked, and half of those who did smoke reported that they had quit. (Probably no other group in society has been more successful in giving up the cigarette habit.) More than 80 per cent said that they were convinced that a cause-and-effect relationship existed between cigarette smoking and lung cancer. Nearly 90 per cent believed that physicians should actively discourage their patients from smoking on general health grounds; 80 per cent believed that their medical organizations should be more active in anti-smoking education; and 70 per cent claimed that they are now engaged, since the Surgeon General's report, in an effort to educate the public concerning the hazards of cigarette smoking, although many doctors were not optimistic about long-term benefits from such campaigns or from such measures as warning labels on cigarettes. Doctors who smoke are less convinced about the evils of smoking than the others, although few doctors would not warn their own children about the habit.

Whether doctors are actually practicing what they preach to pollsters is another matter. As of a few years ago, surveys of patients—as opposed to doctors—showed that less than a quarter of cigarette smokers had ever discussed smoking with a physician, and only one third of these (or 8 per cent of the entire group that had ever smoked cigarettes) had been told by their physicians that cigarette smoking can cause lung cancer. There are, furthermore, few hospitals where one sees posters displayed discussing the hazards of smoking, and there is little evidence that medical staffs have seriously attempted to eliminate the sale of cigarettes from vending machines or canteens on hospital premises.

It is a pity that all insurance companies cannot in some way routinely relate premiums to cigarette smoking. There is evidence that all is not lost even when one has been a cigarette smoker, and that giving up smoking results in lower mortality rates from various causes. A number of insurance companies now do give lower premiums for those who do not smoke cigarettes, even when they do not bother to check up on the truth of a statement to that effect made or signed by the policy holder.

Another ingenious economic incentive has been facetiously proposed by Peter Friedman, an assistant counsel on the Temporary State Commission on the State Constitution of New York. He has pointed out that in view of the 1963 Florida court ruling that the American Tobacco Company could be held liable for death caused by the smoking of the company's product, Lucky Strike, all manufacturers could be held liable for breach of the implied warranty that the product is safe for the use intended. Mr. Friedman states that in order to benefit from such ruling it would be necessary to always smoke the same brand so that "you will know which company to sue. . . . If you take the suggested precautions, you can relax and smoke to your heart's content. When cancer finally strikes, you may rest secure in the knowledge that your cigarette company will provide for your loved ones."

Dr. Howard B. Sprague, past president of the American Heart Association, has written on "What I Tell My Patients About Smoking," and his advice might well be taken by many other physicians. He begins by saying that many of his smoking friends and patients show "a calm heroism bolstered by . . . 'the next guy theory,'" which professes: "Those mortal diseases won't catch up with me. Look, not everyone who smokes dies of cancer, heart disease, emphysema, or bronchitis. I am willing to gamble that it won't happen to me."

Dr. Sprague's first office rule is to set an example for the patient. He allows no smoking in the office, and if a patient tries to light up a cigarette, despite the absence of ash trays, Sprague remarks that the smoke is irritating to him.[1] Occasionally, it is enough to tell the patient that if he stops he will feel better, since many a chronic cough has ceased after several weeks' or months' abstinence from cigarettes. Dr. Sprague occasionally indulges in grisly firsthand tales of the dangers of smoking, especially in an effort to check smokers with peripheral vascular disease, who run a high risk of gangrene, amputations, and death. He finds that statistics are only mild spurring factors by themselves, but useful in conjunction with other exhortations. Finally, Sprague points out that it is terribly important to convince the spouse of a patient that both husband and wife must stop smoking. The smoking of cigarettes around the house by another person is as likely to encourage a chronic smoker to abstain as is the ready availability of heroin to keep a dope addict "clean."

AN AREA OF PREVENTIVE MEDICINE about which the medical profession is understandably ambivalent is the periodic health examination. This concept was first set forth by an English physician, Horace Dobell, in a monograph published in London in 1861. A generation later, an American ophthalmologist named Gould advocated similar examinations in an address before the AMA. Officially, American medicine generally promotes the notion that periodic health examinations are an excellent weapon in the fight against disease. The periodic health examination is based on the premise that supposedly well adults have a great many diseases or propensities toward disease, and that these can be discerned early by a physician. It further assumes that early recognition can lead to prevention, arrest, or cure of a disease, providing the patient is receptive and able to follow the correct advice and action. A good many

[1] Dr. J. Wesley Edel has another approach. He posts notices reading: "Smoking permitted—at your own risk."

adults do have diseases that can be detected, ranging from defects of their teeth, feet, and eyes to matters of malnutrition, syphilis, active tuberculosis, and diabetes. What is not so clear is just how much such early recognition can affect morbidity and mortality and even whether patients will take advice given them on the basis of such screening. Years ago, at the Johns Hopkins Hospital, thousands of patients had routine X rays of their stomachs. Only a few gastric cancers were picked up, and these patients refused surgery because they felt well! In addition, there is a limited capacity to deal with many diseases, so that detecting some illnesses may be meaningless to the patient. Thus it is important to diagnose glaucoma, but arteriosclerosis is at present basically untreatable.

An alternative would be to encourage "early sickness consultation"—that is, patients would be encouraged to see a doctor promptly when they are ill, or think they may be. It has been suggested that such an approach, plus a program of periodic, selective mass-screening techniques utilizing automation and other methods not requiring physician services, might provide as much or more benefit than is now available from periodic health examinations.

Dr. Gordon S. Siegal of the Division of Occupational Health in the Public Health Service has expressed the opinion that periodic health examination of adults remains, after fifty years of vigorous American promotion, a scientifically unproved technique. He points out that we do not have conclusive evidence that populations undergoing such periodic examinations live longer or healthier or happier lives because of it. Siegal believes that the concept has found favor among American doctors because it fits in with the traditional personal doctor-patient relationship, and enjoys popularity because the concept seems reasonable, because the public holds the medical profession and their recommendations in high esteem, and because Americans are a wealthy, health-conscious, and hypochondriacal nation.

If we are to rely on patients consulting doctors for early symptoms, we must ask why patients seek out medical aid. Individuals with sudden serious trauma cannot avoid seeking a physician, but for many complaints, there is unwillingness to consult a physician, and this reluctance is not necessarily related to the seriousness of the condition. Thus for many patients cigarette cough is a "normal" occurrence and not a reason to consult a doctor. Obesity is not likely to be viewed as an illness by patients. Individuals with heart disease or cancer may delay in seeking medical aid because they view the disease as incurable and therefore avoid a doctor so as not to find out the truth. This problem deserves the increased attention of both the lay public and the physician. There is no point in knowing what to do about a disease if the disease is not brought to the doctor's attention or is brought to his attention too late.

It is generally agreed that one of the truly important screening techniques is that for cervical cancer in women. The use of the Papanicolaou smear is of great importance in eradicating this disease, yet many women do not seek such tests. Women with more education and from higher income and occupational classes, as well as those who are convinced that professional judgment is better than self-diagnosis and that the early diagnosis of cancer is beneficial, are more apt to ask for smear tests.

The horror of cancer almost certainly keeps people from discussing it and from seeking medical aid for symptoms that might be caused by malignancy. About 60 per cent of the adult population feel that a patient who knows he has cancer will keep it to himself and not tell others that he has the disease. The most frequently cited reasons for this reticence are that it would turn people away, and that cancer is associated with suffering, disfigurement, operation, incurability, and death.

The statistics on cancer mortality are indeed not reassuring. For most cancers we have drugs of limited power, and if the tumor is not eradicable by surgery or X ray, there is little chance for cure. As already indicated, the mortality trend for lung cancer is upward. So is the trend for a lot of other cancers, except cancer of the stomach, which has decreased for unknown reasons. After half a century of propaganda advising women to seek treatment for breast lumps, the mortality rate from breast cancer remains essentially the same. The data on lung cancer are contradictory. In some series, it appears to make little difference whether a tumor in the lung is picked up by periodic X-ray examinations in the absence of symptoms or whether patients seek advice because they are ill. In other studies, there seems to be an advantage in detecting asymptomatic lung cancer, but patients who come in with symptoms of brief duration do worse than those with symptoms that have been present for longer periods. Findings like these have given some scientists a fatalistic attitude toward most cancers, with a conviction that the prognosis must be determined by the intrinsic biological characteristics of the tumor, the course of which is at present essentially unmodifiable by man.

THERE IS AN ABUNDANCE of health hazards that come from the environment. Some are at least theoretically preventable. Doctors have particular cause for concern about radiation. It is now accepted that members of the medical profession who are exposed to excessive amounts of radiation suffer for it. The most dramatic consequences are skin cancer and leukemia, but recent studies have suggested a nonspecific life-shortening effect of radiation that is reflected in increased mortality from cancer, cardiovascular and renal disease, and indeed all other causes of death. One encouraging aspect of the analysis is that no excess mortality was observed among radiologists in the age class of thirty-five through forty-nine years over the period 1945–58, suggesting that the hazard may have been controlled by recognition of its existence and steps to decrease the exposure of doctors to X rays.

An important question is whether there is much harm inflicted on patients by exposure to X rays during the course of ordinary medical practice. Experiments on both fruit flies and mice reveal no threshold dose for radiation damage. In other words, even the smallest amount of radiation may be genetically harmful, and there is a cumulative effect from exposure over one's lifetime. The fetus is extraordinarily radiosensitive, but the risk to the older individual seems small as compared to other hazards of everyday living. The magnitude of the genetic risk to the population as a whole is not clear. It would appear important to exclude all unnecessary radiation (such as the now outlawed fluoroscopy to fit shoes) and to limit the areas of the body included in exposure during necessary X ray examinations, particularly the gonads. In a Baltimore study, mothers of mongoloid children were found to have had a significantly increased exposure to both fluoroscopic and therapeutic irradiation during the years before the birth of the mongoloid child. These data suggest that maternal exposure to ionizing radiation may be responsible for some cases of mongolism.

Potential mothers are exposed to radiation in programs designed to pick up tuberculosis in individuals unaware that they have the disease. In certain communities there are ordinances that require schoolteachers of the staff of day nurseries to submit annual evidence that they have been examined for tuberculosis. While the goal behind these programs is admirable, one may question the way in which the programs are executed. Screening for tuberculosis can be done by X ray or by the use of the tuberculin test. The latter method is good and eliminates the need for chest X rays of any kind if the subject in question is tuberculin-negative.

But there are also several ways of having one's chest X-rayed. A full-sized regular chest X ray is more sensitive in the detection of early lesions and also provides the minimum of exposure to radiation. Another technique is to use miniature films of various kinds, which are cheaper but not as good in quality, and which, depending on the modernity of the equipment, may subject the patient to as much as ten times the amount of radiation required to take an ordinary chest film.

A different type of environmental hazard exists in the air we breathe. Those who believe that concern about pollution of the atmosphere is a modern phenomenon should read the treatise entitled *Fumifugium or, The Inconvenience of the Aer, and Smoake of London Dissipated* written by John Evelyn in 1661. Evelyn warned King Charles II that the lungs of Londoners as well as their trees would suffer from the smoke that was even then polluting the London air. The warning fell on deaf ears, as it generally does today.

Studies in the United States, Great Britain, and Japan have demonstrated a relationship between the degree of atmospheric pollution and the incidence of respiratory ailments. The occasional local disasters that are reported result from the interaction between a susceptible population (usually people with respiratory or cardiovascular diseases in the old or very young age groups), a lot of industrial and automotive pollution, and a climatological condition such that inversion[2] commonly occurs. More than a dozen such disasters have developed as a result of inversion lasting for three days or longer. The most serious occurred in London in 1952, when in a one-week period there were 4,000 more deaths than normal for the city in that week. There were similar disasters in Pennsylvania in the 1930's, and in New York City in 1953.

Several factors combine to block effective action against atmospheric pollution. There is a certain amount of admitted confusion about exactly what things in the atmosphere cause

---

2 An inversion is said to occur when there is hot air on top and colder air on the bottom (the opposite of the usual state of affairs) with the hot air acting as a lid on the material collecting in the air over a given community. Inversions tend to occur at hours when there is a general tendency for air flow or wind speed to be at its lowest.

harm, and at what concentrations. Absence of unequivocal evidence has been taken by some to mean that nothing can be done until precise information is available. A second factor is the resistance of industrial firms and of automobile manufacturers and drivers to take steps to prevent pollution. It is common—almost traditional—to have industrial representatives constituting a majority of the members of state boards concerned with air pollution. Predictably, such boards often decide that there is no problem from air pollution or that there is a problem but that nothing can be done about it.

Most important, the public is not sufficiently aroused. It may require one or more American disasters comparable to the London tragedy to force effective action at the national level. There is discussion of atmospheric-pollution control, but what is needed is action—legislative and executive machinery to apply adequate pollution-decreasing measures. The public must be made to realize that all human activities that disperse waste into the air must be taken into account and that since air pollution problems do not respect political boundaries, collaborative efforts are required at state, national, and international levels.

The medical profession can help in a variety of ways. There is need for research on animals on the mechanism of harm from atmospheric pollutants. There is need for careful epidemiological surveys to correlate atmospheric pollution and the occurrence of various specific diseases in communities. There is need for the elaboration of realistic standards for clean air. There is probably an important need to study multiple factors, since environmental pollutants almost certainly act in concert with smoking habits, previous cardiorespiratory disease, viruses, bacterial infections, and so on. Most pertinently, the profession must take the lead in educating the public about the hazards and in pushing for realistic controls.

Another environmental hazard in which the medical profession and the public both have interest is noise. The most clear-cut danger is to the ear. As long ago as 1886, T. Barr described boilermakers' deafness in the proceedings of the

Royal Philosophical Society of Glasgow. It is widely accepted now that when there is continual exposure during working hours to noise of greater intensity than eighty-five decibels in any band in the speech frequency range, there may be permanent damage to hearing.[3]

What is less clear is what the effect of noise as a stress may be. Its effect has not been consistent in experiments where work has been measured under conditions of varying degrees of noise. It is even more difficult to state what the emotional effects of noise are, since distress from noise can be as acute from a dripping tap as from a jet engine.

An interesting recent suggestion has been that presbycusis, the loss of hearing thought to be associated with aging, may not be an inevitable concomitant of age, but rather the result of the "cacophony of modern civilization," according to the otologist Dr. Samuel Rosen. Dr. Rosen and his associates made excursions to the bush country of southeastern Sudan to study a tribe of Africans living in virtual isolation. The environment is almost noise-free, having a noise level lower than that of the average home refrigerator in the United States. There is no manufacturing industry or automobile traffic. The tribe has few cattle and little other domestic livestock, and even such rare sounds as cock-crowing are dampened by earth and foliage.

With increasing age, the percentage of these tribesmen able to hear tones of 12,000 to 24,000 cycles per second is higher than that of other groups. In the age bracket from seventy to seventy-nine years, 53 per cent of the tribesmen responded to tones of 14,000 cycles per second, as compared with 2 per cent of those tested in New York City. In general, these tribesmen in their seventies hear as well as twenty-year-old New Yorkers.

To those who have had their sleep disturbed by motorcycles roaring through the street at three o'clock in the morning,

---

[3] Rock 'n' roll addicts should know that amplified guitars and chord organs can produce peaks of 120 decibels.

it is difficult not to feel that noise can be an environmental stress conducive to anxiety and tension, acute or chronic. It may be difficult to prove, but the problem is one deserving of study. Someone has observed that in certain psychiatric hospitals in parts of the world, a purposeful attempt is made to create an atmosphere of peace and quiet. Monasteries traditionally strive to achieve such an atmosphere. Perhaps civilization in general would benefit from quiet.

Such problems as auto deaths, radiation, smoking hazards, air and water pollution, environmental noise, pesticides, and nuclear weapons represent the ability of man to modify his environment at the risk of his health. Man has been slow to develop an ecological conscience, a concern with what he does to affect animals, fish, plants, insects, soil, air, water, and himself.

In developing this conscience man will have to think in larger terms than he has thought before. With his present fantastic abilities to travel, to produce powerful chemicals, and to manipulate nuclear energy, the problems of almost any part of the world become our problems. Dumping sewage into a stream may cause trouble only to a community, but dumping radioactive wastes into the seas may disturb everyone now on earth, and future generations as well. We have to contend not only with airplanes spraying a few million acres with pesticides, but with nuclear blasts that may set the very atmosphere aflame. We may realize, on a global scale, Habakkuk's bleak vision:

> . . . *the fig tree shall not blossom*
> *And there shall be no spring on the vine;*
> *The labor of the olive tree shall fail,*
> *And the fields shall yield no food.*

These threats to man's health have one thing in common—they are all easier to prevent than to correct. The traditional role of the doctor is that of the healer. It will not be easy for him to modify this role, but it is doubtful that he and society can afford for him not to.

Part II

THE QUICK AND
THE DEAD

5

Who Shall Live?

MAN HAS EXISTED on this planet for approximately a million years. During most of this time, he survived by killing the beasts of the field, catching the fish of the sea, and plucking the fruits, nuts, and roots of the plant world, meeting each day's needs as they arose. Under the primitive conditions of this moment-to-moment survival, the world probably never contained more than 10,000,000 human beings. Suddenly—two centuries are, after all, only an instant in the story of mankind—the earth's population began to increase at a frightening rate.

From the time of Christ until the middle of the seventeenth century, the world population doubled. It doubled again in about two centuries, and then again in less than a century. At our current rate of growth, the population would double every thirty-five years. In some lands the population is doubling every two decades. Had the present rate existed since the time of Christ, there would now be 20,000,000 persons for every one now alive—or 100 to each square foot!

In 1965 the Committee on Population of the National Academy of Sciences—National Research Council predicted that if present fertility and mortality trends persisted, "in 650 years there would be one person per square foot throughout the United States. In the very long run, continued growth of the ... population would first become intolerable and then physically impossible."

Is mankind doomed to a relentless physical and mental squeezing that will render life a prison from which death will provide welcome release? What has produced the population explosion? Can it be stopped?

The first cultural mutation to change the status of man dramatically was the invention of agricultural technology some 10,000 years ago. For the first time, several thousand men were able to inhabit an area of land that could formerly support but one person, and human population densities started the gradual rise that preceded the more astonishing changes of the last two centuries. Urban civilizations began to emerge, as a small percentage of men in the society were freed from the tyranny of inefficient, time-consuming hunts for food.

The deforestation of western Europe and the creation of large quantities of arable land followed the availability of the iron ax. On the heels of the Agricultural Revolution came a second revolution, sparked by the new-found ability of man to harness the energy of fossil fuels to run his machines. The Industrial Revolution in Europe was accompanied by an astounding increase in population, although it is difficult to describe the contributory factors with accuracy, since adequate health records were not kept.

Before 1800, the margin of births over deaths was apparently small. Many babies were born, but many died at an early age from infectious diseases. After 1800, birth rates in Europe remained high for more than half a century, but mortality rates plummeted. The two factors probably most important in dropping the death rate were the rising standard of living during the Industrial Revolution and the introduction of sanitary measures about the middle of the nineteenth century.

Infectious diseases that receded in importance during this

time included tuberculosis, typhoid, cholera, scarlet fever, and smallpox. Mortality from tuberculosis began to fall a generation before the other major infections, despite the absence of specific curative or preventive therapy. Some possible explanations that have been proposed for the decline of the "white plague" are that the tubercle bacillus became relatively innocuous, that genetic selection bred out many of those susceptible to tuberculosis, or that crowding—known to facilitate the spread of many communicable diseases—decreased in the home or at work. None of these, however, is thought as likely a cause as the improvement in diet that accompanied the general rise in standard of living.

Cholera, dysentery, typhus, and typhoid diminished because of the sanitary revolution. Water supply and personal cleanliness both improved noticeably, with the expected decrease in incidence of diseases spread by contamination of food and water or by body vermin.

Scarlet fever deserves separate consideration. This fascinating illness has exhibited mysterious cyclic severity in a manner apparently independent of environmental changes and in the absence of specific measures for its prevention and treatment. The changes are probably attributable to the fact that prevalent strains of the causative organism—the hemolytic streptococcus—have varied greatly in virulence.

The body of knowledge that constituted medical science in the early part of the nineteenth century could provide a specific measure to affect the course of only one disease, smallpox. This was the practice of vaccination, which had an impact on smallpox much like that of the Salk and Sabin vaccines on poliomyelitis in the twentieth century.

In our own century, Western countries have witnessed little reduction in mortality rates in middle and later life, although there has been a reduction in infant mortality. In England, for example, 150 of every 1,000 children born in 1900 were dead within a year. The most recent figures show that only 20 of every 1,ooo children now die in their first year of life.

During this period, the developing countries of Asia and Africa have just begun to reap the benefits of public-health measures long available to Europe and the United States. As a result, the changes in mortality rates that began in Europe two centuries ago have been telescoped in time. Whereas it took seventy years to halve the death rate in England and forty years in Japan, Ceylon accomplished this feat in seven years. Meanwhile, birth rates in these new countries have remained relatively high, since education and the use of contraceptive techniques have lagged behind sanitary engineering and the control of infectious diseases.

As a result, these lands are now faced with problems as drastic as they are immediate. Their approach to population control cannot afford to be leisurely. Densely populated, low-income lands are not only faced with permanent trapping at low income levels but must worry about famine. It has been estimated that 1o,ooo people starve to death every day.

It is obvious both that we could feed many times the earth's present population and that food shortages exist. Some of the reasons for this paradox are economic. Hydroponics— the soilless growing of higher plants in water culture—is a technique that can grow much food on little land, but its use has been delayed by the large initial investment required and the higher returns available from non-food-producing enterprises that compete for investment funds.

But there are also less rational factors at work. Many people would rather starve, for example, than change their traditional diet so as to include available items such as insects, rodents, fungi, or seaweed. Africans die every day of kwashiorkor, a disease caused by protein deficiency, but they still object to mixing into bread a tasteless fish flour that could provide the needed animal protein but unfortunately discolors the bread.

Some time ago the Institute for Nutrition for Central

America and Panama developed a high-protein formulated food for small children, to capitalize on the high yield of protein from oil seeds. Meal produced from soybeans, cotton seeds, and peanuts, for example, has a protein content of 50 per cent, as compared with 11 to 12 per cent for winter wheat and 8 to 9 per cent for corn. Despite data showing that children with protein deficiency could be cured by a formula of cotton-seed flour, corn and sorghum flour, yeast, and dehydrated leaf meal, most of the people to whom the product has been introduced (with the exception of Guatemalans) have not been willing to change their dietary habits so as to include the product. Similarly, India produces more than 2,500,000 tons of peanut and cotton-seed meal a year, but undernourished Indian children do not benefit; it is mostly used as livestock feed and fertilizer.

There are many ways by which man could theoretically increase the efficiency of his food production. Acreage currently devoted to food crops could be partly converted to chemical, microbial, and forest products. Control of plant disease and pests might conceivably double our present harvest. A substantial increase in useful food could be achieved, without the addition of any more arable land, by the use of adequate fertilizer and water.

Unfortunately, agricultural techniques that work miracles in temperate zone fail to work in the tropics, where most of the world's hungry people live. Many tropical crops do not respond well to fertilizers. New plant varieties introduced into the tropics fail to thrive, and even when they do, years must pass before enough seed is harvested to plant substantial acreage. Imported cattle are vulnerable to diseases carried by tropical insects.

Some experts have alleged that if one third of our oceans were scientifically cultivated, one third of our total protein requirements could be obtained from fish alone, and possibly a lot more if we wanted to harvest the plankton. The present annual catch of fish could be trebled or quadrupled, even using conventional methods. Seaweed could add 50 per cent to present meat production if it were fed to livestock or used as a soil conditioner. Cattle can be raised without giving them protein of any kind; cows have been successfully reared on ground corn-cobs, synthetic urea, and a little molasses. The bacteria in the cow's first stomach convert almost any form of carbon, oxygen, hydrogen, and nitrogen into amino acids. Cows fed such foods do not give much milk, but the milk they do give is normal, as is their beef.

Hydroponic cultures can yield as much as sixty tons of potatoes per acre per year. Cultures of algae can do double duty, rendering sewage innocuous at the same time they provide food for livestock. An enormous productivity potential is available among certain microorganisms. Under optimal conditions for cell division, for example, one half ton of yeast can synthesize more than fifty tons of protein in twenty-four hours. It has been said that in the time it takes a thousand-pound cow to make one pound of protein, a thousand pounds of micro-organisms can make more than a ton of it.

Not only imagination but know-how is needed by those who wish to achieve the goal of increased food production. Is such a new agricultural revolution likely, and how much will it help the world's population problem?

Why doesn't India, for instance, with a large land mass, grow twice as much food as it does, simply by applying modern agricultural techniques? The answer is that it could—if it had a source of phosphate rock, and plants for making sulfuric acid to treat the phosphate rock, and coal for energy, and plants for fixing nitrogen, and enough trucks and trains to get the fertilizer to the farmers. In other words, a full-blown industrial society is needed in order to apply modern agricultural techniques.

Similar problems apply to the production of milk or fish food. Milk is perishable, and to use it efficiently requires processing plants, which are usually lacking just where they are required most. It has been estimated that to give everybody in this world one cup of milk daily, we would have to build, equip, and open one good-sized milk-processing plant each day for ten years. Fish is also perishable, and large catches must be processed as caught.

In the United States, the growing of broiler chickens has been revolutionized in the last twenty years. Whereas in 1945 it took 4 pounds of feed for each pound of chicken, in 1965 it took only 2.3 pounds of feed. But how is an underdeveloped country to apply the high-energy feeds, antibiotics, pest controls, vaccines, etc., required for such a performance?

It is also apparent that abundant food will not alter the fundamental threat of the population explosion. The growth of a population usually increases exponentially—i.e., fairly rapidly at first, with a plateau later—until environmental resources begin to be in short supply. This is true for bacteria, and seems true for man. If you take an experimental population whose growth curve has begun to flatten out because of limited food supply, however, and provide additional food sources, a new cycle of growth begins, and new population highs result. In short, an increased food supply stimulates population growth.

A quarter of a century ago the Rockefeller Foundation staged a well-conceived and well-executed program in collaboration with the government of Mexico. Far-ranging educational and research measures did indeed produce substantial increases in food production. Yet after two decades, the population increase had outdistanced the increase in food, so that everyone had a little less to eat than before.

Physiological changes in man correlate with food supply in a way that would support this general contention. In the presence of severe food shortage, menstrual periods are disturbed or stop, and fecundity is seriously affected. This was seen in Holland during a six-month famine period in 1944, in Nazi concentration camps, and during the siege of Leningrad in

World War II. More subtle, but still important, effects occur even in the absence of such severe deprivation. The poorer the living conditions in a community, for example, the higher the proportion of stunted women. Such women have pelvic abnormalities that cause difficult labor, force Caesarean section more frequently, and lead to higher perinatal death rates from birth trauma and other causes.

Is it possible that similar "corrective" medical effects or genetic selection may help solve our population explosion? Some animal species seem to utilize mechanisms for restricting population size that, in a complicated and not thoroughly understood manner, control the amount of space available for each member of the species. Forty years ago, a small herd of deer was placed on an island in the Chesapeake Bay and kept well supplied with food. The colony grew rapidly until it reached a density of one deer per acre. Then the animals began mysteriously to die off, despite adequate food and care. Autopsies revealed changes in the adrenal glands in response to the stress of crowding, and there were a variety of physiologic consequences, including reproductive failure. It has been postulated that the deer had, via slow evolutionary change, selected out genes that made them suffer when they encountered one another too frequently. This usually forced them to keep their distance, but for the deer on their new island home there was no escape.

Man, however, seems unlikely to show similarly drastic reactions to crowding. Those who by genetics or acquired taste show a preference for isolation will probably become extinct while those who welcome or tolerate high population densities thrive. While it is certain that excessive human crowding causes physical and mental hazards, we must remember that in a place like Hong Kong, people manage to survive at a density of 12,700 per square mile.

While adequate food will thus not solve the population problem, and may indeed aggravate it, sustenance is nevertheless required for the earth's increasingly more numerous inhabitants. One wonders how many people our planet could conceivably support. Harrison Brown, Professor of Geochemistry at the California Institute of Technology, has answered the question in this way:

> If you were to make me Dictator of the World I could support 200,000,000,000. I could, provided people did what I told them to do. . . . I might have to ask them not to move around. They would have to lie on their backs; be stacked up on shelves some place. I would feed them very efficiently—entirely on vegetable matter, naturally. I might occasionally give them a steak, which I would make out of alfalfa curd. . . . I might put some plastic sinews in it to make it chewy. . . . It would be pretty expensive, and pretty difficult, but I am sure our engineering genius would enable us to feed 200 billion people. I am not saying you would be comfortable; I'm just saying I could feed you. . . . You would exist.

Some have argued that things are not as black as they seem. The United States birth rate, for example, has declined steadily since 1958. In 1935, at the depth of the depression, 77 babies were born per 1,000 American women of childbearing age. By 1957 it was 123, a forty-year high. (It had been around 275 in 1800.) But since then the rate has steadily declined, so that it is now less than 100. In fact, 1965 was the first year since 1953 that the total U.S. births did not reach the 4,000,000 mark.

This decline is not, as one might think from all the publicity about oral contraceptives, simply due to "the pill," which was not in significant use in the United States until 1961–2. The Public Health Service has suggested some possible explanations. First, the proportion of fertile women (i.e., the percentage aged fifteen to forty-four) has declined over the last twenty-five years. Second, there has been a drop from the unusually high birth rates in older women during the 1950's, when couples were presumably making up for births postponed during the late 1930's and early 1940's. Finally, there has been a drop in birth rate among younger couples, partly because of a tendency to space births more widely, and partly because smaller families are now more desired.

In Great Britain, a similar fall in birth rate began unexpectedly at the end of 1964 and has continued through 1966. The Russian figures parallel those in the United States, and the rates in Bulgaria, Czechoslovakia, Hungary, Poland, Rumania, and Yugoslavia began to fall even sooner and have dropped at a faster pace.

In terms of population density, the United States is still a thinly populated nation, with 50 persons per square mile. Switzerland has seven times as many people per square mile, and the Netherlands more than seventeen times as many. Even with a population density of 300 we would still have less people per square mile than present-day Italy, West Germany, the United Kingdom, and Japan.

Countries such as Mexico and Guatemala continue to record high birth rates, and India and China together probably produce close to 40,000,000 new infants each year. At the 1965 meeting of the United Nations Population Commission, expert demographers concluded that the world's population would probably double to 6,000,000,000 by the year 2000 even if the two thirds of the world not now practicing family planning began to reduce their birth rates. The gloomy soothsayers would seem more realistic than the optimists.

To make matters worse, the problems discussed thus far have not even included the auxiliary ones that automatically come with population growth. More children mean more schools, more houses, more clothes, more hospitals, more jobs. As Sir Theodore Fox has pointed out:

> To say that a country will have another 10,000 children next year may seem a small matter; but, just to maintain its previous educational level, that country will have to build, equip, and staff a new school for 400 children every fortnight, which certainly will not make it any easier to reduce the size

of classes and improve the quality of teaching. In India 10 years ago fewer than 40 per cent of children were at school, and one wonders what the proportion will be when the school-age population has risen to the 150 million predicted for 1978. These will be the parents of the next generation; and, if they remain uneducated, not only will they be too primitive to be an effective labour force but they will also preserve the traditions of early marriage and excessive childbearing. Breeding yet more people.

When these additional children are educated, they will need employment. In the United States, it has been estimated that a job in industry is now capitalized at between $50,000 and $100,000. In Puerto Rico, during its first eight-year period of intensive industrialization, the cost per job averaged $6,400 and in recent years has risen to $20,000. Mexico estimates a need to put 390,000 people to work each year between now and 1980. If this could be done for $10,000 per job, it would require an annual capital expenditure of nearly $4,000,000,000, a huge sum for a country that lacks capital. In fact, a new Mexican polyethylene plant that employs only 200 workers cost more than $8,000,000, a capitalization of $40,000 per job.

Kenneth E. Boulding, Professor of Economics at the University of Michigan, has pointed out that a high rate of population growth must be accompanied by an equally high rate of growth in the nation's capital in order to "stand still." Thus a society with 3 per cent annual increase in total population must increase its capital stock annually by 3 per cent, and if capital stock is twice its annual income, that society must save 6 per cent to achieve progress and development. But it is just the big family that will have a difficult time accumulating any savings.

Most people would agree that we must focus not on the problem of achieving a world that is as crowded as possible, but one in which individuals can live with sufficient dignity and privacy to preserve the spark of humanity. John Maynard

Keynes once asked: "Is not a country overpopulated when its standards are lower than they would be if its numbers were less?" *At some point in time, then, population growth has to stop.* This means a choice between increasing death rates and lowering birth rates. The first is repellent to most, whether it involves famine, plague, war, or euthanasia, and the second is distasteful to some. But there are no other alternatives.

In seeking methods to control the size of the population, there is at present overwhelming preference for the individualistic approach. While some religions prefer to consider one's body as belonging to God, man acting merely in the role of a tenant, there is a growing sentiment in favor of the philosophy that a person should control his own body and its functions. Logically extended, this means the moral legitimacy of contraception, and indeed of abortion. It means free access to all methods of population control as a human right, and the deliberate separation of sexual activity and pleasure from childbearing. The National Academy Report quoted from earlier in this chapter asserts: "The freedom to limit family size to the number of children wanted when they are wanted is, in our view, a basic right."

Such views are not only humanistic in orientation, but democratic as well. Yet the basic freedom to plan the size of one's family is not equally available to all levels of society. While the great majority of American couples approve of (and practice) some form of contraception, the poor in general do not. Disadvantaged groups often simply do not have informal sources of information, such as knowledgeable friends or relatives, and seldom consult private physicians for advice. The poor do not so much desire large families as lack the knowledge and means to restrict family size.

Whatever one's point of view about the right of the individual in regard to birth control, there are few who would prefer these decisions to be made by governments. And yet if individuals cannot control the growth of population, governments must someday determine by law who may and may not reproduce, and when. Professor Boulding has speculated on the possibility that someday the government will give adolescents marketable licenses to have children. The price of these licenses, which would be limited in number, would be determined by the market demand. Boulding says the scheme illustrates "the kind of drastic measure that will almost certainly be necessary." The succeeding chapters will discuss some other solutions to the excessive multiplication of man.

6

Sex Without Fears

IT IS PARADOXICAL that man should be plagued by population problems. The human female is a late procreative bloomer, first able to produce offspring somewhere around fifteen years of age. Compared to some protozoa, which start to reproduce a few hours after birth, this is sexual retardation of an advanced degree. Man does not hold the record, to be sure—the periodic cicada is seventeen years old when its reproductive activity occurs and the Sumatran rhinoceros is said, by intrepid students of reproductive physiology, to attain puberty at twenty years— but we are close to one extreme. Herring gulls, bullfrogs, and lobsters need only three to four years to shift into genital gear, and such diverse living things as the pink salmon, the dragon-fly, the yak, and the blue whale can breed when two years old.

The rate of sexual maturation is directly related to the potential of a species for population growth. For man, it is thought by some experts that age at marriage is possibly a more important determinant of future population than is total family size. Species that mature rapidly, on the other hand, such as the passenger pigeon (one year) and the fur seal (three years), are very vulnerable to reduction of life expectancy during the reproductive ages, and a decrease in offspring even from five to four significantly reduces their potential for population growth.

Age also has other important biological meanings. The efficiency with which a woman bears babies begins to decline fairly early after sexual maturity. The incidence of spontaneous delivery in less than twenty-four hours after onset of labor is highest in the fifteen-to-nineteen age group, as is the chance of having a perineum elastic enough to stretch before the infant's head without tearing or without the need for an episiotomy. After twenty-two, a steadily increasing percentage of mothers require assistance to complete delivery for no other apparent reason than that they are unable to expel the baby themselves. With increasing age, there is also a rise in the incidence of unexplained intrauterine death, hypertension, and toxemia of pregnancy.

Most insects—and insects constitute three quarters of the animal kingdom—can be classed as annuals, since they mature and reproduce in a single year. So, too, do some mammals, birds, fishes, and amphibians. All species that produce offspring singly must of course reproduce at least twice in a lifetime to avoid extinction. The human female, which averages 0.5 female offspring per birth and has a gestation period of 280 days, is a contender for the record low reproductive potential. Compare the ameba, which can divide in two every couple of days; the female housefly, which can produce 200 eggs and go through eighteen generations per year; oysters, which produce about 60,000,000 offspring per year; or the busy tapeworm, which can pass 120,000 eggs per day for decades.

Despite recent concern with the population explosion, man has apparently tried to control the growth of his species throughout his social evolution. The history of organized, planned efforts to help the masses acquire a knowledge of contraception is only a century or so old, and the achievement of reliable contraception is quite recent, but the desire to control births has characterized most societies, even those whose religious codes have admonished people to "increase and multiply."

In preliterate societies, contraception has never been the chief population control. Early checks were rather of the death-producing variety—epidemic diseases, famine, war, human sacrifice, and natural catastrophes. In primitive societies, probably the chief birth-limiting check has been abortion, a topic to be discussed in a later chapter. Other preventive measures included delayed marriage and celibacy (not very popular or effective), sex taboos, sex perversions, pre-pubertal coition, prolonged lactation.

Conception control in such cultures was probably both magical and rational, and elements of both persist in the customs of present-day primitive peoples. Some African tribes abstain from normal intercourse upon birth of a child, beginning again when the child starts to crawl. During this period they do not practice total continence, but rather coitus reservatus or interruptus. Other tribes use crushed roots as an intravaginal plug. In South America, native women have been reported to insert an okra-like seed pod five inches long, with one end snapped off, into the vagina, thus producing a vegetable condom. Such rational techniques were presumably arrived at by trial and error, since the physiology of conception is not well understood in such societies.

In striking contrast are the magical methods. In northern Africa, a small leather bag, in which is sewn a Koranic formula, was worn around the waist to prevent pregnancy. In Morocco, corpses were believed to have a sterilizing effect, so that women anxious to avoid pregnancy would linger behind after a burial and step three times over the grave. Water used for washing a dead person was given secretly to women to drink, to render them infertile. In eastern Africa, women seek out knot-tying experts, who search out two kinds of bark in the woods. These are twisted into a cord, into which is rubbed the yolk of an egg. Three knots are tied while incanting a curse of sterility. To undo the curse, the woman has to untie the knots, place the cord in water, and then drink the water.

Recommendations in those ancient Egyptian records available to us include a nauseating concoction, presumably intended for insertion into the vagina, of crocodile's dung mixed with a paste of some sort. The famous Ebers Papyrus of 1550 B.C. refers to a medical tampon consisting of lint moistened with honey and the tips of the acacia shrub. These tips contain gum arabic, which can be transformed to lactic acid, a chemical used in the United States and Britain as an ingredient in contraceptive jellies.

In the Book of Genesis is told the story of Onan, whose sin consisted not of masturbation, but of refusing to impregnate his brother's wife and practicing coitus interruptus with her. The rabbis proclaimed such practice a mortal sin, despite the fact that other religious leaders recommended coitus interruptus when it was medically indicated. Thus Rabbi Eliezer, about 80 to 100 A.D., wrote of the period during which the mother nurses her child: "During the twenty-four months, he [the father] must thresh inside and winnow outside." Catholics view Onan's error to be the practice of birth control, whereas others tend to believe that the Lord slew Onan for refusing to adhere to the law of the Levirate.

The authors of the Talmud seemed aware of the possibility of using a moistened sponge, placed in the vagina before cohabitation, to cover the uterine opening and absorb the semen. Possibly such a practice—later recommended by Francis Place in nineteenth-century England—was derived from the Egyptian lint tampon, knowledge of which could have been acquired by the Hebrews during their captivity. An interesting idea that the ancient Hebrews shared with primitive peoples concerned the contraceptive benefits of violent motion. Violent contortions of the body after cohabitation were supposed to prevent insemination.

Many Greek and Roman writers touched upon the population problem. Hesiod, Xenocrates, and Lycurgus favored the one-child family. Plato wanted the age of procreation to be limited by law to thirty to thirty-five years for men and twenty to forty years for women. Aristotle would have had the number of children per family legally limited, and he approved both abortion and the slaying, by exposure, of deformed infants.

Pliny the Elder, in his *Natural History*, has some weird ideas about how to dampen sexual ardor. His anaphrodisiacs included mouse-dung liniment, nasturtium, hemlock applied to the testes at puberty, and a potion of willow leaves. He reported that if a woman's loins were rubbed with blood taken from the ticks upon a wild black bull, she would be averse to sexual intercourse. (The risks taken by the modern drug industry and pharmacist are obviously minimal when compared to the derring-do required of Roman potioneers.)

Aëtios, a Greek physician of the sixth century, mentioned washing the male genitals with vinegar or brine—spermicidal substances used in modern times as douches. Aëtios, like other ancients, was unacquainted with douching, but he could go down in history as a pioneer with the right thing at the right time but in the wrong place, were it not for the fact that vaginal douching is probably little more effective than the technique he espoused.

Rhazes, called the greatest physician of the Middle Ages, had some interesting advice for the planned-parenthood federation of East Baghdad:

> . . . the expulsion of semen from the uterus may be effected in several ways. Firstly, immediately after ejaculation, let the two come apart and let the woman arise roughly, sneeze and blow her nose several times, and call out in a loud voice. She should jump violently backwards seven to nine paces. . . . the woman may sit upon the tips of her toes and squeeze and rub her navel with her thumb. She may smell foul odors or fumigate her under parts.

Then, in one of the great anticlimaxes of all time, the Persian genius added: "Joking too is useful."

Casanova, the great lover of the eighteenth century, apparently not content to kiss and tell, had more than a passing interest in birth control. One technique he described consisted of cutting a lemon in half, extracting most of the juice, and using the disk as a cervival cap. He also favored the use of an intravaginal gold ball, testifying to fifteen years of satisfied use:

> It is sufficient for the ball to be at the base of the temple of love when the loving couple carry out the sacrifice. . . . But, says the friend, movement may displace the ball before the end of the libation. . . . This is an accident which need not be feared, provided one exercises foresight.

The condom represented an important advance in the history of contraception. Many primitive peoples, as well as the early Egyptians, used various forms of penis protectors, not for contraceptive purposes, but for such diverse reasons as modesty, decoration, status symbols, amulets to promote fertility, and protection against diseases and insect bites.

The first known published description of the condom is found in Fallopius's *De morbo gallico*, published posthumously in 1564. The author, a distinguished Italian anatomist, described a linen sheath, which he claimed to have invented. He praised it with a testimonial in which he cited its successful use by 1,100 men to prevent acquiring syphilis: "I call immortal God to witness that not one of them was infected."

Madame de Sévigné, in the seventeenth century, had some reservations about condoms—or at least against a sheath made of gold-beater's skin which she dismissed as "armor against enjoyment, and a spider web against danger."

The very word "condom" is of uncertain origin. Some claim it to be derived from one Dr. Condom or Conton, a physician at the court of Charles II. One idea had it as stemming from the name of a French village in the department of

Gers. Another related it to the Latin *condus*, the substantive of the verb *condere* (to conceal, protect, preserve). Another theory traces the term back to a Persian word referring to a long vessel made of the intestines of animals and used to store grain. Neither of the two European nations most often related to its development seem to want credit: the French call the condom "the English cape" and the English call it "the French letter."

Casanova knew and used the condom, referring to it at various times as "the English riding coat," "the English vestment which puts one's mind at rest," "the preservative sheath," and "assurance caps." He apparently used condoms both to prevent infection and to avoid impregnating his lady friends, and is said to have tested the condoms for imperfections by inflating them with air.

The founder of the modern birth-control movement was Francis Place (1771–1854). A self-taught workingman, Place was the first to make an organized attempt to educate the masses in the use of contraceptive methods, as opposed to Malthus's advocacy of "moral restraint." Place's prime propaganda weapon was the handbill. As methods he recommended coitus interruptus and the intravaginal sponge. His exhortation was oriented mainly to the prevention of poverty and raising the standard of living, although he did mention contracted pelves and constitutional weaknesses. Place also believed that birth control would bring about earlier marriages, and thus reduce vice, prostitution, and venereal disease. There was no legal interference with his early propaganda, and thousands of handbills were distributed. Although there is no convincing evidence that Place's campaign had an immediate and measurable effect on the British birth rate, it almost certainly helped to set in motion other similar social efforts.

In America, the birth control movement was begun around 1830 by Robert Dale Owen and Charles Knowlton. Owen, who considered birth control inevitable, recommended techniques similar to those espoused by Place. Knowlton's chief reliance was on douching with cold water, alum, tea, plant extracts of various kinds, or baking soda.

Late in the nineteenth century, contraception received considerable impetus from two famous trials. The first involved two Freethinkers, Charles Bradlaugh and Annie Besant, who decided to test the legality of selling a Knowlton pamphlet after a man named Henry Cook and his London publisher, Charles Watts, were convicted of selling the pamphlet interleaved with obscene pictures. Arrested and tried before Lord Chief Justice Cockburn, Annie Besant and Bradlaugh, an able lawyer, collaborated brilliantly to win the case. The publicity attending the trials was tremendous.

The second case concerned the aged and esteemed Freethought publisher Edward Truelove, whose issue of two tracts on birth control brought down on his head first the wrath of the Society for the Suppression of Vice and then the police. After one trial, which ended in no verdict, Truelove was sentenced to four months in prison and a fine of fifty pounds. Liberal and radical circles denounced the Society for the Suppression of Vice, and when Truelove was released at the end of his prison term, he was met by a rejoicing, celebrating crowd.

Meanwhile, millions of people had learned that contraception was possible. Prior to 1876 Knowlton's "The Fruits of Philosophy" had sold about 1,000 copies annually. In the three and a half years after the Besant-Bradlaugh trial, 185,000 copies were sold of just one edition, while other editions swelled the sales to over a quarter of a million copies. From 1880 to the present time, the proponents of birth control have waged an irregularly successful battle to make contraceptive information available to all who desire it.

Gradually, new contraceptive techniques were introduced and old ones improved. Large-scale use of the condom became possible after the invention of the vulcanization of rubber. By

1882, the German physician Wilhelm Mensinge had devised the vaginal diaphragm, which became, until a decade ago, the contraceptive device most often prescribed by American private physicians and birth-control clinics. Spermicidal creams, jellies, and foams were introduced. In the 1930's, Kyusaku Ogino in Japan and Hermann Knaus in Austria independently developed the rhythm method, based on the fact that the ovum is released from the ovary about two weeks before the onset of the next menstrual flow.

Then, in the late 1950's, the contraceptive pill arrived. On its heels came renewed interest in intrauterine devices. Both techniques were hailed as revolutionary by some and roundly condemned by others. How they were developed, how well they work, and how safe they are will be discussed in the next two chapters, but in order to appraise them accurately, it is necessary to examine first the relative popularity and effectiveness of other modern contraceptive techniques.

In 1955, just before the advent of the oral contraceptives, a national study of birth-control methods found the great majority of American women favoring three techniques. About 25 per cent relied on male use of condoms, 25 per cent preferred diaphragms, and another 25 per cent used the rhythm method. This represented a considerable change from the situation two decades earlier, when the vaginal diaphragm was rarely used, the modern rhythm method was just being described, and the condom shared top honors with withdrawal and the postcoital douche.

It is estimated that 4,000,000 to 5,000,000 gross of condoms are sold each year in the United States. (Sales in France are thought to total 150,000 gross. Even when you correct for the smaller French population, it still comes to only one condom per adult French male per year as opposed to a dozen per adult American male.) A highly efficient electronic method of quality control has been developed to monitor condom production. Except for drawing each sheath by hand over a cylindrical metal mold, the process is completely automated. As a result, one worker can test more than 2,000 condoms per hour. A conveyor belt carries the condoms to a tank of water that contains a surface-tension-reducing agent. The mold and the tank are electrically charged, with only the condom barring passage of current. If current is observed to flow, the sheath is removed from the production line and destroyed as scrap. (Apparently 10 to 15 per cent are so eliminated.) Condoms surviving this trial by electricity are dried, stamped, rolled, and packaged.

In addition, the U.S. government interposes further safeguards between the trusting consumer and pregnancy by defect. The Food and Drug Administration spot-checks interstate shipments and periodically inspects condom factories. Samples drawn at random are subjected to a water-leakage test. Each condom is filled with ten ounces of water, twisted at the end, and then rolled over a dry towel to detect leakage. In practice, most defects are manifested by a thin jet of water during the filling of the condom, but to detect very small holes requires that the condoms be rolled on a towel or filter paper. These procedures apply not only to the domestic output of U.S. manufacturers, but also to the products imported into the country for domestic use. (We seem to take no official notice of condoms headed from American shores for foreign use.)

Such quality-control measures have produced gratifying results. In 1934–5, 2,149 sheaths, representing twenty-one U.S. condom brands, were tested, and 60 per cent were found defective. Today, less than 0.5 per cent are found defective. By contrast, in a 1963 water-leakage challenge of British condoms 3 to 12 per cent, depending on the brand, flunked the test. (Although the prices of these condoms varied over tenfold, there was no clear correlation between quality and price.)

When carefully used, condoms are associated with low pregnancy rates. Such rates are lowest—as with many other methods—among couples with the highest incomes; in this group the rates are about as low as with most other available techniques. The major cause of failure is rupture of the sheath. "Pinhole" defects are thought to be relatively unimportant, since only a small amount of semen can escape via this route. Careless withdrawal of the penis after detumescence may also cause escape of semen. Despite the occasional failures and the psychological and mechanical barrier to uninhibited sexual satisfaction, this technique remains a popular one, especially in casual sex situations.

Another extremely reliable form of contraception is the vaginal diaphragm, which needs to be fitted by a skilled physician, so that its use is initially contingent on medical intermediaries. Its successful use requires that it be inserted either daily as a bedtime routine or before each intercourse, so the method is not for those lacking in diligence. Rare failures occur even with regular use, and are thought to be attibutable to dislocation of the diaphragm and subsequent insemination during the vaginal expansion that accompanies sexual excitement. This occurs most often in women who have already had children, those who engage in a sequence of repeated coitus over a period of hours, and those favoring the female-superior position.

Various creams, jellies, tablets, and foams are used separately or in combination with the diaphragm. All of these contain or liberate chemical contraceptives that immobilize sperm on contact, and they also provide a mechanical barrier of sorts. It is almost impossible to say with precision how good such materials are, primarily because there have been almost no controlled experiments that would enable comparative statements to be made with assurance. Despite the fact that population-control experts seem to recognize that the performance of contraceptives is highly affected by such variables as motivation, socioeconomic status, age of the partners, and duration of use, researchers who plan clinical trials cavalierly disregard these factors.

As a result, anything desired can be proved by picking the "right" scientific articles from the medical literature. Failure rates for contraceptive jelly, for example, vary fivefold in published papers. One can examine a pair of studies and conclude that the diaphragm-plus-jelly technique is five times superior to foam tablets, or a different pair and conclude that the tablets are twice as good as the diaphragm-jelly combination. Even the same data have been analyzed to yield strikingly different conclusions: one set of authors reported one pregnancy rate for a new contraceptive cream jelly, whereupon another expert recalculated and concluded that the true figure was at least four times higher. If the players on the field are confused, what of the poor spectators? The best guess I can make, after inspecting the various reports, is that the cream-jelly-foam-tablet approach is far superior to the vaginal douche, but not as safe as the condom or diaphragm.

Coitus interruptus and withdrawal are still more risky, as well as psychologically frustrating, but are utilized by some couples whose religion proscribes mechanical or other devices. In this group, also, fall the adherents of the rhythm method.

The notion that the human female is infertile during part of the menstrual cycle is an old one. The Greek gynecologist Soranus, who lived in the second century A.D., recommended avoiding intercourse right before and right after menstruation for women wishing to prevent conception. As late as 1883, this same advice was still being given. Since such a regimen will help achieve conception, not prevent it, it is understandable that the approach fell into disrepute.

Independent Japanese and Austrian work in the 1930's finally set things straight, taking advantage of the knowledge that the ovum is released from the ovary about two weeks before the onset of menstrual flow. Because of the substantial irregularity in many women's menstrual cycles, abstinence for the ten days clustered around midcycle is the minimum requirement for success, and the safe period during which intercourse is allowable is restricted even further if there is marked menstrual irregularity.

Body temperatures measured in the morning before rising are higher during the second half of the menstrual cycle, but the rise is less than 1°F. and is not easy to detect in all women. Furthermore, since the rise occurs one or two days after ovulation, its most useful function in contraceptive technique is to suggest when sexual relations can be resumed. What would be truly helpful is either a test that would give a dependable signal three days before ovulation, or a way to induce ovulation on a given day. Research is being conducted along the latter line with hormones and chemicals.

The rhythm method is admittedly far from optimal, although if carefully used it deserves better than the scornful epithet "Vatican roulette." It is important primarily for Roman Catholics, since their church formally sanctions only this method of fertility control. Before the oral contraceptives —about which individual priests and church officials have disagreed—perhaps half the Roman Catholic couples in the United States relied on rhythm, while the others used methods considered illicit by their religious leaders.

In some ways the most important aspect of official approval by the Catholic Church of the rhythm method is its acknowledgment that sexuality as such is an important value in married life, and does not exist solely for procreative purposes. The development of this attitude harks back to an extraordinary fifteenth-century professor at the University of Paris, Martin Le Maistre. An eclectic, he drew skillfully on both Aquinas and Aristotle. His position was radical for the times, rejecting Augustinian doctrines. "I say that someone can wish to take pleasure, first for the love of that pleasure, secondly to avoid tedium and the ache of melancholy caused by the lack of pleasure. Conjugal intercourse to avoid the sadness coming from the absence of venereal pleasure is not culpable." Maistre's theses were espoused by a sixteenth-century Scottish theologian, John Major, who stated: "Whatever men say, it is difficult to prove that a man sins in knowing his own wife for the sake of having pleasure." During the centuries that followed, the idea that pleasure was a proper end in marital intercourse was increasingly supported by prominent Jesuits, Dominicans, and secular priests, and the position was common after 1900. The future will in all likelihood see further revision of Catholic doctrine to allow a more modern approach to human passions.

The biologist Garrett Hardin once tried his hand at writing a second Sermon on the Mount. One of his beatitudes was: "Blessed are the women that are irregular, for their daughters shall inherit the earth." He went on to explain:

> The rhythm method is, when used by women who have a rhythm, only two and a half times as bad as "artificial" methods. . . . But even if it were every bit as good, it would be self-defeating. For there would still be those arrhythmic women, about one in six, for whom the method is meaningless. Compelled by dogma to reject artificial methods, these women would soon outbreed the rhythmic ones. If there is even a tiny hereditary element in their irregularity (as there surely must be), natural selection would then ultimately produce a world populated only by irregular women.
> Tidings of Darwin should be carried to Rome.

7

Procreation, Profits, and Paralysis

THE MOST controversial population-control development of the century has been the oral contraceptive—the pill. From its impeccably scientific beginnings, the pill has become all things to all people—spelling riches and fame for some, sexual security to many, and death for a few. Among scientists, it has inspired both religious zeal and grave suspicion.

The original observations were made in the 1930's, when it was found that natural sex hormones inhibit ovulation in animals. Male and female hormones were both observed to block ovulation but were not thought suitable for clinical use because of concern about either their effectiveness or their side effects, although sex hormones were used to treat painful menstrual cramps, which do not occur in nonovulating women.

In 1954, Carl Djerassi applied a new chemical technique to the synthesis of different steroid drugs, some of which were shown to be orally effective progestogens—substances that produce secretory changes in the endometrium similar to those produced by progesterone. Gregory Pincus tested 200 of these in animals and found three to be very powerful inhibitors of ovulation.

A few years earlier, Professor John Rock of Harvard had treated infertility in women with daily doses of estrogen and progesterone to simulate the hormonal environment of pregnancy, during which there is growth of the uterus and Fallopian tubes. The continuous hormonal therapy eliminated menstrual periods, a phenomenon the patients found disturbing. As a result, it was decided to give the hormones only from day 5 to day 25 of the cycle, and thus allow menstrual flow. Rock, Garcia, and Pincus proceeded to use this same regimen with the three active oral compounds mentioned above, but now to prevent conception, not achieve it.

In most cases, ovulation was inhibited, as witnessed by changes in the lining of the uterus and vagina, in hormone excretion, and in the appearance of the ovaries in the few women who were examined for this at the time of abdominal surgery. Large-scale field trials were begun in Puerto Rico, and the pills were a great success in terms of both contraception and patient acceptability. A few years later, after additional experience in the United States, the Food and Drug Administration approved the sale of the first contraceptive combination of estrogen and progestogen, Enovid.

The mechanism of action of these preparations is still debatable. Inhibition of ovulation is probably the most important effect, but the lining of the uterus is also rendered unsuitable for implantation of the egg, and the consistency of the cervical mucus is maintained in its nonovulatory, relatively impermeable state.

How effective is the pill? The medical and lay literature contains a good many quotations from different scientists to the effect that the pill never fails "if taken according to instructions." Critics of this euphoric assessment point out that failures with the pill tend to be attributed to inability to follow directions even when the women swear that they never forgot a single daily dose. They also emphasize that if a technique fails because of human error, it is a failure nevertheless and must be considered part of the risk. It is also disturbing that many women in studied populations drop out of the study; there is no way of evaluating the pill's performance in these possibly disenchanted women.

It is unreasonable to expect perfect performance from the pill. With all drugs, there is variability in response to a given dosage, due to vagaries of absorption, metabolism, excretion, or organ response, so that what works well for one patient may not work well for another, or even for the same patient at different times. One method of diminishing such variability is to give everyone a dose that is known to be an overdose for some. This is done with penicillin in the treatment of pneumococcal pneumonia. The reason for not adopting this approach routinely with all drugs is that it also generally increases the chance of producing side effects from the drug. This is not a serious problem with penicillin, but it is with oral contraceptives, and has led to a good deal of manipulation of dosage. As the dosage has been reduced, some side effects have apparently diminished—and, incidentally, the cost of this still-expensive form of birth control has been reduced. It seems predictable that some patients will get pregnant while taking the pills even if they are compulsively careful with their dosage, and this number will probably be higher as the dose per day is reduced to diminish unwanted effects. (There is at present no evidence that such pregnancies will result in malformed babies more frequently than will other pregnancies.)

Nevertheless, even those who are least enthusiastic about the pill grant its excellent performance as a birth-control technique. If the risk of pregnancy is not zero when taking daily oral contraceptives, it is very low indeed. Nor is this the only advantage. It is easy to use—just a pill a day. It does not have to be timed to intercourse. Its use does not delay, interrupt, or mechanically impede the sexual act. It is attractive to many men and women who object esthetically to condoms, diaphragms, jellies, and foams. Finally, some Roman Catholics who reject other devices against which Church officials and parish priests have been less equivocal in their denunciation are willing to take the pills.

The customary vigor of American pharmaceutical advertising soon led to public clamor for the pill. From 20,000 U.S. users in 1957, the number rose to 1,400,000 in 1963, with at least a further doubling since then. Its use is also widespread in other countries. By 1965, half of the young married women in Australia were said to be taking some form of oral contraceptive. Many manufacturers, eager to cash in on the tremendous market, introduced competing products. Some of these were "me-too" products, but a few manufacturers have tried to be more imaginative. Several "sequential" products are now available, which claim to be "more physiological." With these, the estrogen component is taken alone for fifteen days, followed by estrogen and progestogen together for another five days. Unfortunately, there are reports suggesting that any advantages offered by products of this type in terms of side effects may be offset by a greater risk of pregnancy.

A recent step is the use of infrequently spaced medication. At least one contraceptive seems to work well when injected only once per month, and plastic capsules have been devised that are implanted under the skin and slowly release hormone for years. Dr. Robert B. Greenblatt at the Medical College of Georgia claims success with a pill taken only once a month. The clinical experience with this method is limited, and to date its use has been associated with considerable nausea and prolonged bleeding.

In *Cosmopolitan* for July 1965 appeared an article entitled "Oh What a Lovely Pill!" It promised women that "a honey of a hormone, properly used" could "end menstrual pain and the ravages of the menopause, act as a contraceptive or increase fertility." One devotee of the pill was quoted as saying: "I'm going to take these pills all my life. I wouldn't dream of giving them up. Even when I no longer need birth control pills, I'll

take them just for the difference they've made in my health
and my responsiveness to my husband."

The claims made for this modern snake oil are impressive.
Do you have acne? Take the pill. Dysmenorrhea? Take the
pill. Avoid the menopausal syndrome? Take the pill. Prevent
heart attacks, strokes, overweight, diabetes, skin wrinkles, kidney troubles, cancer of the breast or uterus? Take the pill. The
author admitted that "lifelong therapy does not mean that
women will be forever young" but asserts that they will be
"forever feminine," with healthier hair, smoother skin, firmer
breasts, a finer figure, and a higher mattress rating. Sad to say,
there is little or no convincing evidence to back up most of
these claims.

The Mahatma of this Mini-Menopause is a Brooklyn
doctor named Robert Wilson. His book *Feminine Forever*
sold more than 100,000 copies in its first six months in the
stores, although an AMA book reviewer commented that "by
offering unattainable benefits . . . Dr. Wilson . . . is taking
advantage of a most susceptible group of women." He has
attracted the FDA's attention because some of his assertions
extend the claims for oral contraceptives beyond the approved
labeling. (The pills have never been approved to prevent the
menopause or cancer; in fact, the pills are not supposed to be
taken by a woman suspected of having breast or genital cancer.)

Dr. Wilson's research is supported by the Wilson Foundation, a tax-exempt organization formed in 1963 "to foster,
promote and support research investigation in all phases of
cancer research." Except for the secretary and one other person, the board is a family affair: Wilson, his wife, his son, and
his son's wife. Most of the foundation's funds have come from
contraceptive manufacturers—Ayerst, Searle, and Upjohn.

The foundation's activities are said to be largely educational. It invites queries about treating the menopause, mails
free medical literature to women and doctors, provides lectur-
ers and films to women's clubs, and has obviously been highly

successful in planting stories in popular magazines. Whether it has done the American female a service or not is less clear. Estrogen therapy has for years been used to treat flushes and other menopausal symptoms or to prevent or treat menopausal bone-thinning, but most doctors would not share Dr. Wilson's belief in the miracles he claims. Wilson—who has treated everyone from convent nuns to a seventy-two-year-old English-woman whom he put on a crash program to ready her for her wedding night—is undeterred.

The picture has not been all rosy with the oral contraceptives. From the start it was obvious that the pill had drawbacks. Some women gain too much weight. Others develop acne, nausea, vomiting, or breast tenderness. More distressing are such things as sporadic breakthrough bleeding, depression, excruciating headache, tension, decreased libido, loss or excessive growth of body hair, skin pigmentation, and belly or pelvic pains. Some lactating mothers stop producing milk and have to resort to artificial feeding for their babies. Newer oral contraceptives have claimed a decreased incidence of these various side effects, but none of them is free of nuisance potential.

Most frightening of all, thus far, has been the occurrence of clotting within the blood vessels. In 1961, fatal pulmonary embolism occurred in two young Los Angeles women who had been on oral contraceptives. Next, women on the pill were observed to develop thrombophlebitis as well as clots that traveled to the lungs. Since then, all sorts of clotting troubles have been reported in women taking the pills. Thrombosis of the blood supply to the gut, with gangrene of the intestine, has been seen. Thrombosis of the major arteries in the arm and leg has been reported, requiring amputation. A London physician observed strokes in a twenty-three-year-old airline stewardess and a twenty-six-year-old housewife. His report prompted a Sussex physician to describe two similar cases and to state that he knew of at least three others. A Newcastle physician announced that the autopsy on one of his young women on the pill showed clots in the arteries on both sides of the brain.

In April 1965 the Johns Hopkins neurophthalmologist Frank Walsh asked his fellow specialists (via the *Archives of Ophthalmology*) to report to him any cases they had seen with visual troubles similar to those he had observed in women on oral contraceptives. By November he had assembled some sixty cases in this way—seventeen with strokes, twenty-one with eye troubles, and twenty-three with other symptoms, including migraine. Without claiming a cause-and-effect relationship, he nevertheless wished to put the experience on the record and to ask for further study.

Meanwhile other physicians continued to report deaths as a result of compromise of the blood supply to the nervous system. One twenty-six-year-old Englishwoman died of a clot in her vertebral artery after a seven-week illness during which she had paralysis of all four extremities. In Ireland, a twenty-five-year-old patient expired with a large dead area in her brain caused by a clot in the carotid artery.

Dr. Sherif Shafey in Miami was at the same time accumulating his own series of thirty-four women, ranging in age from twenty to thirty-nine years and all receiving some form of oral contraceptive, who developed various sorts of neurologic complications, including migraine headache and clots in the arteries and veins of the brain.

Next, effects on the heart were reported. In January of 1965 a Norwegian pathologist described the sudden death of a thirty-two-year-old woman who had been taking oral contraceptives for five months. Postmortem examination revealed that the smaller branches of the coronary arteries were plugged with clots of various ages, with resulting death of the heart tissue. This was followed by a fatal case from England with clots in all of the major arteries of the heart, and others have since been recorded.

Why have these cases been put on record by physicians from various parts of the world? All the complications described are known to occur in people who do not use oral contraceptives. No new diseases have been seen. Why, then, the concern over the possibility of a cause-and-effect relationship?

It must be remembered that the suspicion of alert physicians is almost always the first indicator of pharmacotherapeutic mischief. Rarely can the doctor do more than suspect a cause-and-effect relation between drug and toxic effect, since hardly any drug's side effects are unique to that drug. Further, massive pulmonary embolism, strokes, and heart attacks are relatively rare in young women. This is a recurrent theme in the statements of concerned physicians, such as the British doctor who wrote:

> This cause of death [pulmonary embolism in a twenty-two-year-old woman on oral contraceptives for a few months] . . . in young people is extremely rare. In the few cases I have seen in young women there has always been some underlying explanation. . . . It is this feature which has been worrying me in my examination of an otherwise perfectly healthy woman. My own feeling is that [it] is just too much to be a coincidence. I have never seen a similar case . . . and I have seen many unexpected deaths in young people. This does not amount to proof.

Supporting this sentiment was a letter from a Cambridge scientist:

> From 9280 consecutive autopsy reports . . . covering 1946–63, we have collected 27 cases [of massive pulmonary embolism] under the age of 70. Of 21 . . . females, only 3 women were under the age of 45, and they were either pregnant or had recently been pregnant. Thus we have no examples of non-pregnant women . . .

Other studies are in agreement. The coroner's records of Cuyahoga County in Ohio were reviewed in 1964 to see how often pulmonary embolism and unexpected sudden death occurred in supposedly normal persons between fifteen and forty-five years of age. Sixteen females had died in this manner during an eleven-year period. Five of these were pregnant at the time of fatal embolism, and eight of the eleven nonpregnant females were over forty. Thus, while such unexplained deaths are not unheard-of in young women, they are decidedly rare.

In Hamburg, Germany, a study was made of fatal pulmonary embolism in a series of 5,200 autopsied cases. Of 500 consecutive cases of pulmonary embolism, half were in women, but their average age was seventy, and 95 per cent were over fifty.

A few cases have shown such unusual autopsy findings as to alert doctors to a generalized clotting tendency. In one case autopsied at the Johns Hopkins Hospital, for example, there were numerous clots in arteries and veins all over the body, without any actual disease of vessel walls.

But there are other compelling reasons for suspecting the oral contraceptives as a causative factor in these vascular catastrophes. Many of the scientists who have worked with the pill have compared the endocrinologic state induced by these synthetic steroids with pregnancy. While this view is not universally held, there are at least certain parallelisms between normal pregnancy and drug-induced pseudo-pregnancy. As stated above, pregnancy carries with it a definite risk of clotting difficulties, related in part at least to the hypercoagulable state associated with the hormonal alterations undergone by the expectant mother. Both during pregnancy and the taking of oral contraceptives, there is also a reduction in blood-flow velocity in the extremities, which favors the formation of sludge in the vessels of the limbs.

Although the pill buffs tend to ignore them, a substantial number of studies have now been performed to determine whether oral contraceptives affect the clotting capacity of the blood. They have been conducted in such diverse places as Oslo, Norway, and Manchester, England, and in the United

States in Washington, D.C., Minneapolis, Brooklyn, Philadelphia, New York, and Seattle. The majority agree on the fact that there are changes from the normal, even in asymptomatic women taking oral contraceptives. These scientists have not all used the same tests, but in general there have been increases in blood factors II, VII, and X, and fibrinogen (the precursor of fibrin, which eventually forms the clot). Blood platelets, in the two studies focusing on this blood constituent (which helps clots to start), were also increased in number. Only one index of blood clotting—the so-called fibrinolytic system—possibly changes in a direction that might impede normal clotting. *All the other changes are such as to encourage the clotting of blood.*

There are other reasons for worry. In several studies in men and women who have been given female sex hormones as treatment for atherosclerosis of the brain or heart, or for cancer of the prostate, there have been significantly more deaths in the treated patients than in the control (untreated) patients, with more strokes, heart attacks, or both.

Studies of blood fats have shown changes in women on the pill that resemble those seen in post-menopausal women, who have a higher risk of heart attacks than younger women. One extremely provocative report involved a Mead Johnson oral contraceptive that was under trial in 7,000 American women. Trials were suddenly halted when British workers giving "massive doses . . . daily and continuously for several months" to dogs reported thromboemboli in the animals.

A number of researchers have been intrigued by the relationship between hard-water areas and the decreased occurrence of hypertension and other cardiovascular diseases. It has even been suggested that a diet deficient in magnesium may be partially responsible for the high incidence of arteriosclerosis in Western nations. In 1966, Drs. John and Naomi Goldsmith reported serum magnesium concentrations to be lower in non-ovulating women and women on Enovid than in ovulating women. The finding calls only for speculation at present, but it supplies another bit of evidence to remind us of the multiple effects of hormonal agents.

With such highly suggestive data, how can one explain the unwillingness of many physicians even to consider the possibility of clotting troubles in some women taking oral contraceptives? One major reason for this apathy is the now famous report of the 1963 Advisory Committee asked by the FDA for guidance in evaluating thromboembolic morbidity and mortality.

The committee decided to focus only on fatal complications, because of the difficulty in tracking down nonfatal cases. (A patient whose lungs were riddled with clots and who survived only because of heroic cardiopulmonary surgery, or who suffered a disabling but nonfatal stroke, thus did not enter into their deliberations.)

It was necessary to know how many women had died while on Enovid, the drug under investigation. For this purpose, they relied completely on the files of G. D. Searle, the manufacturer. This was the first and most appalling mistake. No drug manufacturer can possibly have complete records of the deaths occurring among patients taking his drug. To have such complete records would require that every such death be associated in the attending doctor's mind with the possibility of its being caused by Enovid, that he always know whether patients have been on Enovid, and that he report every such case to the manufacturer. All experience is contrary to these assumptions. Even in hospitals where drug reactions theoretically must be reported by the medical staff, and simple cards are provided for such purpose, the true incidence of drug toxicity varies from ten to fifty times the incidence calculated from what is voluntarily reported.

The committee also relied on photostats of death certificates for knowledge of what was occurring in the population at large. Regrettably, death certificates are notorious for their inaccuracies, especially when autopsies are not performed. As Professor L. M. Schuman, a member of the committee, said on a later occasion: "In view of the fact that one of the greatest sources of error in hospital statistics is the glib assignment of a clinical diagnosis to pulmonary embolism . . . epidemiological studies utilizing mortality sources should confine themselves to autopsy-confirmed material."

There was also no clear information on how many women were taking the pills. It was known roughly how many prescriptions had been filled and renewed for Enovid, and after some crystal-ball gazing, it was decided to subtract 300,000 (primarily to exclude duplicate prescriptions) from the maximum estimated numbers of users to give a tidy—but possibly inaccurate[1]—figure of 1,000,000 women. No one on the committee seemed to worry, however, about the fact that it was important to know not only how many women took Enovid during a given year, but also how long they were on Enovid. (A lady on for only one month is obviously not at risk from the drug for the whole year; to assume so is to make the drug look safer than it is.)

Next, the committee decided to throw out some of the Enovid deaths, for a variety of reasons. Unfortunately, such selective discarding of cases could be done easily for the Enovid cases, but not for the control group. The latter were studied only by analyzing death certificates, whereas the Enovid files contained autopsy reports, clinical information, charts, etc., solicited by the manufacturer or voluntarily supplied by the reporting doctor.

There were many other assumptions as well, but these are perhaps the most disturbing. What, then, could anyone conclude from such an analysis? Nothing, of course, which is what the report actually says:

There is a need for comprehensive and critical studies regarding the possible effects of Enovid on the coagulation balance and related production of thromboembolic conditions. Pend-

[1] The number of women on the pill has been a subject of controversy. In 1966, for example, it was first guessed that 6,000,000 women were on it, then 5,000,000. A private survey by the National Fertility Study indicated 3,800,000.

ing the development of such conclusive data and on the basis of present experience this latter relationship should be regarded as neither established nor excluded.

Unfortunately, the report also included the statement that "no significant increase in the risk of thromboembolic death from the use of Enovid in this population group has been demonstrated." The FDA, the pill enthusiasts, and most physicians have since then acted as if the report, which is based on incomplete data of dubious quality inappropriately analyzed, actually proved for all time that there was no risk.

This attitude has been encouraged by several other factors. The manufacturers of Enovid, for example, have periodically informed the world that the cases reported are not in excess of those "anticipated." In 1965 their medical director published a paper with the astonishing news that the thromboembolic morbidity was actually less than a quarter of what might have been expected. He conceded that the discrepancy "is very likely a reflection of inadequate reporting" but concluded with the unequivocal assertion "that massive use of Enovid has not increased the incidence of thromboembolic disease in women."

A second source of misconception is the group of experts who for one reason or another have decided that the pill's advantages must not be sullied by any doubts. One argument is that pregnancy is risky too and that the troubles women get into on the pill must be balanced against the medical risks of pregnancy. Such an argument is reasonable, of course, only for those women who cannot possibly use any other effective contraceptive technique.

Dr. Erik Ask-Upmark, head of the Department of Medicine at the University of Uppsala in Sweden, reviewing his own and others' experiences with thromboembolism in women on oral contraceptives, pointed out the highly suggestive recurrence of trouble in several women as they took repeated courses of pills. His report ends: "If any female member of my own family applied to me to get oral contraceptives I would most certainly not dare to give it to her."

In 1965, a WHO Scientific Group came in with their own report. There was a certain friction in the committee, especially from an American expert who bridled at the need—spelled out in WHO rules—for unanimous recommendations. The report pointed out that incidence of thrombophlebitis is highest not in pregnant women, but right after delivery, when hormonal levels are lowest. This was meant, presumably, to exonerate the pill, which is said to produce a "pseudo-pregnancy." It might be argued, however, that women on the pill have a "pseudo-delivery" once a month, as they suddenly stop the pill in order to menstruate. (Such an argument presumes that the pill produces a menstrual cycle more like pseudo-pregnancy than normal menstruation.) Recent studies also suggest that much of the clotting troubles seen after delivery are not "spontaneous" but due to estrogens given to suppress lactation in non-nursing mothers.

The report also made an interesting and subtle point: many doctors will not prescribe oral contraceptives in women with a history of thromboembolic disease. Thus in a sense the pill is being given to healthier women than the average population, possibly biasing present risk estimates in favor of the pill. The committee concluded that oral contraceptives were extremely effective and that no cause-and-effect relationships had been established for serious adverse effects. Nevertheless, it listed twenty unmet research needs, including the effects of the pill on the pituitary, "higher nerve centers," thyroid, adrenals, carbohydrate metabolism, ovaries, cancer development, genetics, uterus, vagina, lactation, infants, liver, blood, weight, emotions, congenital anomalies, and a variety of diseases!

In 1966, the Food and Drug Administration came up with still another report on oral contraceptives. Unfortunately, the expert committee was no more able than its predecessor to make factual statements about serious risks from the pill. It acknowledged that deaths from thromboembolism were of concern, and that "the present system of reporting deaths and adverse reactions relies on either the cooperation of physicians or the haphazard filtering of rumors to detail men. The latter route is patently unreliable, and the former not much better. Physicians are becoming increasingly fearful of reporting deaths or adverse drug reactions because of possible legal reprisal." (I know of two deaths in Baltimore—from strokes in twenty-one- and twenty-six-year-old girls—unpublicized for this very reason.) The report reiterated that available data could neither confirm nor refute the role of the pill in thromboembolic disease. No progress, in other words, since the 1963 FDR report.

The committee expressed worry about the carcinogenic effects of estrogen taken for long periods, admitted that long-term studies to tell whether the pill might cause cancer were unavailable, but concluded that no maximum limits should be set for how many years the pill might be taken.

Other risks were also discussed, but the important conclusions reached were as follows:

> The committee finds no adequate scientific data, at this time, proving these compounds unsafe for human use. It has nevertheless taken full cognizance of certain very infrequent but serious side effects and of possible theoretic risks suggested by animal experimental data and by some of the metabolic changes in human beings.
>
> In the final analysis, each physician must evaluate the advantages and the risks of this method of contraception in comparison with other available methods or with no contraception at all. He can do this wisely only when there is presented to him dispassionate scientific knowledge of the available data.

Dr. Roy Hertz, a National Institutes of Health endocrinologist and cancer specialist, filed a minority report for the committee that took a much graver view of the pill-cancer problem. He reminded people that all known human carcinogens show a long latent period—most of them about ten years, but ranging up to forty years—and that in most instances there is no way of detecting this fact during the period when the cancer is "cooking," as it were. Hertz also pointed out that all known human carcinogens are also carcinogens in animals and that therefore animal data are not irrelevant, as some have claimed. (It is ridiculously easy to produce tumors of all kinds in rats, mice, rabbits, hamsters, and dogs given estrogen, and early in 1966 an investigational drug of this class under study by Merck Sharp and Dohme was hastily removed from clinical trial when dogs developed breast cancers after a year of treatment with the Merck contraceptive.)

He then reviewed the accepted evidence that a young woman's own estrogen or estrogen in pill form can make breast cancer worse, and observed that most breast cancers are probably in existence for years before they become clinically apparent. Hertz derided the claims that use of estrogens in women over the last twenty-five years had not changed the incidence of breast cancer, because most of the women so treated have not been young women, but were post-menopausal, and there is clear evidence of a difference between these ages in response to female hormones—estrogens are even used successfully to treat breast cancer in older women. He further revealed that the entire world literature on the risk of prolonged estrogen therapy causing breast and genital-tract malignancy is based on a pitifully small sample of less than 1,000 women, of whom only 85 were under forty years of age. He then performed a similar analysis of the worrisome situation with regard to uterine and cervical cancer, and the possible effects on ova and children ultimately born from the eggs of women who have taken the pill. In none of these situations could Dr. Hertz find reason for complacency. He ended with this unequivocal recommendation: "In view of the serious limitations in our knowledge of the potential long-term effects of estrogen-progestogen combinations, it is mandatory that further clinical experience be gained under properly controlled conditions of observation and follow-up."

The FDA report elicited predictable reactions in the interested parties. Physicians suspicious of the pill saw cause for alarm, and found no reassurance. The drug manufacturers saw the report as an exoneration of the drug. Dr. Louis M. Hellman, chairman of the FDA Committee, said the report was a "yellow" caution light. Dr. Alan Guttmacher of Planned Parenthood read it as "a complete green light." One could only recall the story of the blind men and the elephant.

The British at first did no better than the Americans. In a country with a highly organized National Health Service with allegedly good record keeping on drug usage, they relied on voluntary reporting by doctors instead of careful detective work on women in the childbearing years who died of strokes, heart attacks, pulmonary emboli, etc. The results were as inconclusive and unsatisfying as might be expected: "At present the number of deaths [voluntarily] reported is small and does not differ remarkably from expectation . . . [however] the deaths reported . . . may represent an underestimate . . . no firm conclusion can be drawn . . ."

A week earlier, in the *British Medical Journal*, which carried the above report, a distinguished Oxford professor wrote on "Adverse Reactions to Drugs," pointing out that the actual incidence of toxicity with a new drug with which he had worked was twenty-five times higher than one would guess from voluntary reporting by practitioners, and that one could temporarily at least quadruple the reported incidence by sending official requests for information to all British doctors. Obviously the hazards of underreporting are universal, as is the likelihood that official government committees and drug manufacturers will neglect these hazards.

In the spring and summer of 1967, however, three independent British studies were reported that finally began to clarify the thromboembolic danger. All delivered an affirmative answer to the question "Can oral contraceptives cause thromboembolism?" In the words of a Medical Research Council Subcommittee: "The sum of evidence . . . is so strong that there can be no reasonable doubt." It remains to be seen what impact, if any, these findings have on the prescribing habits of physicians.

Although the blood-vessel abnormalities have received the greatest publicity, other potentially serious complications of the pill have been reported. In 1964 some Finnish scientists reported abnormal liver function in seven post-menopausal women who consented to take oral contraceptives for a month. Despite dissents from some experts and manufacturers, there has now been convincing confirmation of this phenomenon in different parts of the world, including the United States, and involving women in their twenties as well as older females. Particularly at risk of developing jaundice are those rare women who develop the unexplained "jaundice of pregnancy," which is probably also attributable to hormonal changes. It is not reassuring to learn that mestranol, present in most oral contraceptives, can cause severe liver damage and even liver cancers in rats taking the drug in high doses for prolonged periods.

Others have observed decreased tolerance for glucose in some women taking oral contraceptives, with "chemical diabetes," a phenomenon again reminiscent of what occurs during pregnancy. Whether this is related to the changes in blood concentration of adrenal or thyroid hormones that occur in women on the pill is not clear.

A few letters have appeared in the British journals describing strange muscle pains or symptoms of neuritis associated with the taking of oral contraceptives, and diarrhea related to structural changes in the lining of the small intestine. American doctors have seen dilatation of the ureters in women taking oral contraceptives.

Gynecologists have occasionally observed severe uterine bleeding in women who have stopped the pill after prolonged cyclic therapy for contraceptive purposes. The bleeding is thought to be due to overgrowth of the lining of the uterus secondary to disturbance of normal feedback mechanisms among the ovary, the hypothalamus, and the pituitary. Other gynecologists have been troubled by the development of an "obstinate" form of vaginitis due to the yeast Monilia in women taking oral contraceptives, curable in many cases only after the pills are discontinued.

Psychiatrists have been upset by the unpredictable mental effects of the pills. Some women on them claim an increase in sexual desire and pleasure, but others become frigid, a situation reversible by stopping the pills and using mechanical devices. Dr. William Masters, co-author of *Human Sexual Response*, said that when referring physicians or marriage counselors ask him to see a woman for secondary frigidity, his first question is: "Has she been taking the pill?" There has been an increasing awareness of depressive reactions, with crying spells or suicidal ideas, in women taking these hormones. Some believe that the pills can make a latent depressive state overt or aggravate an existing melancholia. Remission may not follow promptly on withdrawal of the drug.[2]

Fears about the long-range effects of oral contraceptives on fertility have ranged from apprehension about ultimate infertility when the pills are stopped after years of use to the possibility that oral contraceptives, by preventing ovulation, may prolong the period of potential childbearing so that pregnant fifty- and sixty-year-old grandmas will be possible. One Canadian physician has even suggested the possibility of a new specialty of "geriatic obstetrics" to care for such aged parents. There are no convincing data at present to support either notion, although both American and Australian physicians have suggested some women may suffer long-term interruption of their ovulatory cycling as a result of the pill, with prolonged failure of menstruation (and infertility) after stopping the

2 It must also be stressed that some women, such as those who suffer from severe premenstrual tension, may be helped remarkably by taking oral contraceptives.

medication. Proponents of the pill promptly labeled the reports "misleading" and the conclusions "unwarranted."

In view of all the side effects reported with the pill, and the clear evidence that some 10 to 25 per cent of women refuse to go on with oral contraceptives because of dissatisfaction of one sort or another, it is confusing to have their enthusiasts deny such defects. In April 1966, *The New York Times* ran a "gee-whiz" type of article about the pill entitled "Three Men Who Made a Revolution." In it, Dr. Gregory Pincus commented on the medical advertising for some newer-type sequential and low-dosage pills: "These ads are creating a false emphasis. There may be a minute lessening in side effects, but since all present side effects are insignificant, I see absolutely no advantage in sequentials."

Such a remark stands in strange juxtaposition to the drug ads. One for Ovulen, for example, reads: "A significant advance over older progestins . . . a new measure of freedom from undesirable effects . . . extremely low incidence of breakthrough bleeding . . . low average weight change . . . extremely low incidence of nausea . . . extremely low incidence of amenorrhea . . ." If these statements do not imply a better performance than with older drugs, what are they saying? And if Ovulen is so remarkable, one wonders why the ad explains, in tiny print to be sure, "the following adverse reactions have been reported with Ovulen: headache, dizziness, depression, breast complaints, amenorrhea, chloasma, vomiting, allergy, edema, migraine, pulmonary embolism, thrombophlebitis, visual difficulties, nervousness, rash, itching, decrease in libido, tiredness and malaise. A small incidence of nausea, spotting and breakthrough bleeding has been reported."

What is a sensible, conservative, scientific attitude toward the use of the pills? On occasions when I have taken a public position emphasizing the possible dangers of their use, it has been obvious that the emotions of both patients and doctors are highly charged when it comes to a discussion of oral contraceptives. Doctors have accused me of everything from a Catholic-tainted bias against contraception (I left the Church at the age of twelve) to having canine ancestry on my maternal side. These doctors are understandably annoyed because such discussions upset their patients. But is it really defensible to assure women—as many doctors do—that the pill has been proved as safe and harmless as water? (Nothing is as harmless as water, including water.) How can a doctor say that he "can think of no condition in which these pills would not be safe to take"? (The FDA labeling warns against their use in certain situations.) How can Dr. Rock in an article entitled "Let's Be Honest About the Pill!" dismiss those who worry about its dangers as "irresponsible, and uninformed . . . zealots"? Does he really believe that all women who find themselves unable to tolerate any brand of oral contraceptive on the market are, in his words, "guilt-aroused neurotics"? Is it really desirable to produce diabetes temporarily with the pill because this merely unmasks a condition that would have become manifest years later and is therefore "a prophylactic blessing"? Surely such questions deserve serious discussion, not supercilious dismissal.

These pills should certainly not be taken off the market. On the other hand, they cannot possibly be considered the contraceptive technique of first choice for all women desiring birth control. They are not necessarily the best or the only way. The pills are indicated for many women, including those who will not or cannot use mechanical devices because of anatomic, psychological, or religious reasons. Since it is my firm conviction that these pills can kill—rarely, to be sure—and that other techniques, properly used, which do not kill, are almost as effective in preventing conception, I believe it bad medical practice not to recommend mechanical contraception to those who can use it. I recognize the tremendous importance of the pills for certain women who apparently find condoms and diaphragms impractical despite the great need some of them have for means to avoid pregnancy, and I appreciate the Planned Parenthood Association's interest in avoiding hysterical condemnation of the pill. But it is ethically and morally wrong to take the decision out of a patient's hands by assuring her that these powerful chemicals are completely free of risk.

It has been argued that even if one recognizes some small risk from the pill, its advantages far outweigh the dangers. One Baltimore obstetrician argued that a million women not using any contraceptives would experience 360 maternal deaths per year, since most would become pregnant,[3] and some women die of pregnancy. His guess about oral contraceptives was that a million women taking them would show only one or two maternal deaths, and that a few additional deaths from thrombophlebitis and related vascular troubles would still be acceptable. A main point of his argument is the assumption that use of the condom or diaphragm would result in 50 maternal deaths per year because of a high failure rate with these devices.

How valid is such an argument? Another Baltimore obstetrician, equally well known and experienced, pointed out that the failure rate of the condom or diaphragm—properly used— is very low. The higher figure obtains in couples with low motivation—for example, those who have one child and are not quite sure when they want a second. An excellent batting average is seen in highly motivated women—those who have completed their families, for example, and are sure that they don't want another child. In his opinion, most failures "are simply an expression of 'I don't care.' " And one thing is reasonably certain—condoms and diaphragms are not going to produce breast cancer, or diabetes, or any of the other ills that are at least a theoretical hazard of oral contraceptives, which can affect the whole body, not just the uterus.

It would be wonderful if doctors could predict which women would get into trouble from the pill, but at the moment it is possible only to avoid its use in certain women, such as

[3] They would not, of course, be pregnant every year, however, a fact ignored in the calculations, which also do not jibe with the more recent British data.

those with obvious vein disease, past or present, and a history of migraine or of jaundice during pregnancy.

The pill has raised all sorts of difficult side issues. In Los Angeles Planned Parenthood classes, any girl under the age of twenty-one can have oral contraceptives if she brings in a note from her mother. The rationale is that illegitimate pregnancy is a greater hazard than the possible fostering of promiscuity in teen-agers. This prompted a Connecticut physician, however, to rephrase a story describing this Los Angeles philosophy so as to read: "We will give contraceptives to teen-agers provided the mothers are willing to declare in writing that their daughters are promiscuous." He ended by quoting from Isaiah: "Woe unto them that call evil good and good evil."

In defense of the practice, Dr. Edward T. Tyler, a California expert on population-control methods, pointed out that it is not uncommon to see girls thirteen and fourteen years old first appearing in clinics with full-term pregnancies, bearing children who are unwanted and usually prove a heavy burden to those involved as well as to the state. He also offered to introduce the Connecticut doctor to a Los Angeles minister who requested a branch of the Planned Parenthood Clinic to be started on the premises of his church, but only on condition that its services be dispensed without restrictions as to background, age, or marital status of those requesting the services.

The law courts will soon be busily embroiled in debate over the pill. A talented group of lawyers in New York has been retained by a number of plaintiffs from all over the country for the initiation of litigation against manufacturers of oral contraceptives. These plaintiffs are women (or families of women) who have suffered one or another serious complication of the pills and who are demanding damages. The first such case was entered (and lost) in 1965, but more are sure to follow.

In Brazil, the pill has upset Pan-American relations. The Guanabara Medical Association, along with other Brazilian left-wing organizations, wants to prohibit sale of the pill and other birth-control devices. Their argument is that population control is a subversive extension of U.S. policy, which aims to restrict Brazil's population, and thus its national strength. If the pill has had no other effect in Brazil, it has at least temporarily united the left wing with the Catholic Church—no mean task.

Religion is inextricably intertwined with the story of the pill. The Roman Catholic Church, so closely identified for many years with opposition to birth control, has been re-examining its position in the last few years, but has refused to endorse the pill. Dr. John Rock is himself a Catholic, and in 1963 published a book arguing that since naturally secreting progesterone provides the "safe period" in the rhythm method and during pregnancy protects the fertilized egg from a competing conception, why not utilize a sterility produced by a duplicate of the natural agent, namely the pill?

Cardinal Cushing of Boston chided Dr. Rock for having forgotten the Church law that requires Catholics writing on subjects of faith or morality to submit the manuscript to Church authority for an *imprimatur*. He then dismissed Rock's thesis as failing to meet the basic arguments against his position raised by moral theologians.

The liberal Catholic journal *Commonweal* was upset in a different way by the debate: "Is it any wonder . . . that a book as inadequate as Dr. Rock's should receive publicity out of all proportion to its merits and soundness? Where most Catholics tread with muffled shoes and theologians keep their doubts to themselves, anyone who speaks frankly is bound to be made either a hero or a villain. . . . The time has come . . . to confront anew the issues which he raises." For relatively unbiased non-Catholic scientists, *Commonweal*'s conclusion seemed reasonable enough, since it was easier to agree with Rock's goals than with the mental pretzel-bending required to describe the use of synthetic hormones as a modified rhythm method with a permanent safe period. Meanwhile, millions of Catholic couples continue to choose between unwanted pregnancies, sinning, and sleeping in separate rooms.

8

Silver Rings, Plastic Bows, and Sperm Banks

DESPITE THE GREAT popularity of the oral contraceptives, they are clearly not the last word in birth control. In places as far apart as Mecklenburg County, North Carolina, and Chicago, Illinois, the pill has been given up, for a variety of reasons, by as many as 25 per cent of the women who have tried it. Some of these dropouts, to be sure, are women whose doctors, concerned about possible complications, stopped the medication despite the absence of worrisome symptoms. But more women who give up the pills do so because of unpleasant manifestations, such as nausea, bleeding, or weight gain, or because of an unintended pregnancy. This overall failure rate is lower than that for the diaphragm-and-jelly method, and the efficacy of the oral contraceptives in preventing conception is obviously high, but these experiences show the need for alternative techniques.

The most exciting new development along these lines has

been the resurgence of interest in intrauterine devices. Certain nomadic tribes have for centuries practiced intrauterine contraception at the veterinary level. No Arab (or presumably anyone else) is keen on starting off for a distant goal with a pregnant camel, since apparently a gravid dromedary not only tires easily, but is difficult and stubborn. To prevent pregnancy, a round, smooth stone is introduced into the uterus of the camel, who thereupon repulses the advances of male dromedaries as if she were in fact pregnant.

While there is reference to intrauterine devices in Hippocrates' *Diseases of Women*, their modern application dates to the late nineteenth century. In 1878, intrauterine devices (which protruded from the cervix and served to occlude its opening) were used medically to prevent pregnancy. As early as 1916, Dr. R. L. Dickinson predicted that a pessary wholly within the uterus would one day be adopted as a birth-control technique. German gynecologists led the field in this search, the most well-known being Ernst Gräfenberg. He began in 1928 to publish a series of articles describing completely intrauterine gadgets made of silver, gold, or silkworm gut. His experience, especially with the metallic coils of wire, was thoroughly satisfactory, but others had less luck, especially in regard to complications such as inflammation and infections.

The approach fell into disfavor because of these complications; only one report on intrauterine pessaries was published between 1934 and 1959 in a Western medical journal by any physician who had himself used them. Textbooks of gynecology either ignored the rings or condemned them. Even Gräfenberg, although he never changed his favorable opinion, rarely used his rings after he came to the United States in 1940.

In 1959, however, the medical world was stimulated to take a second look. The Israeli gynecologist W. Oppenheimer published on his twenty-seven-year experience with the use of rings of silver or silkworm gut. His patients had a low pregnancy rate and seemed to suffer no harm. Dr. Atsumi Ishihama, at about the same time, put on record an analysis of Japanese experience with more than 18,000 women, also with highly favorable results.

In 1962, Dr. Alan Guttmacher, who has been president of the Planned Parenthood Federation of America, toured the world to study the birth-control problems of other nations. He returned convinced that the population explosion could only be contained by three techniques—oral chemicals, immunization methods, and intrauterine devices. The first he saw as already being effectively promoted by drug manufacturers. The second would not be applicable for many years, if ever. That left intrauterine contraception, and he recommended that the Population Council concentrate its funds and talents on this third approach.

The council followed his advice and organized a conference attended by representatives from eleven countries. A film on intrauterine contraception was made and shown all over the world. In the next four years the Population Council spent over two million dollars on the project. A comparative study of five different devices was underwritten, and data were collected from hospitals in the United States, England, Fiji, Puerto Rico, Hong Kong, and Sweden. More than 100,000 women were carefully studied in a short period of time. When the second international council on intrauterine devices was held in 1964, there were more than 500 participants from forty-four countries.

Of the modern intrauterine contraceptive devices (IUCD's), three—the Margulies spiral, the Lippes loop, and the Birnberg bow—are made of polyethylene plastic, with an added barium salt that renders the device visible by X ray. Each can be stretched out straight and threaded into a tube with the bore of a soda straw. The straw is then passed through the cervical canal and the device inserted into the uterus with a plunger. Once in the uterus, the devices spring back into their original form. The Hall ring is a coil spring of stainless steel, while the Zipper ring is made of nylon fishing line.

The spiral, loop, and coil have tails that protrude from the cervix and serve two functions. The first is to allow patient or doctor to tell easily if the device is still in place. The second is to facilitate removal of the device. The other IUCD's must be removed with a button-hook sort of instrument, a not difficult task in most women who have previously borne children. The insertion of IUCD's is at present generally performed by gynecologists, but there is no great objection to such insertion being done by trained midwives or nurses.

No one knows for sure how IUCD's achieve their contraceptive effect. In the rat, a foreign body in the uterus does not impede fertilization of the egg, but the eggs disappear after reaching the uterus. In the rabbit, some fertilized eggs actually implant in the uterus, but none develops. In the cow, the egg apparently does not implant. In the monkey, there is evidence —not accepted by all—that the IUCD causes the smooth muscle of the oviduct to become hyperactive, so that instead of a leisurely three-day trip down the tube, the eggs race down in a few hours, like harassed commuters. Either the eggs are not fertilized during this *Blitzreise*, or they reach the uterus so early that they, the tissues lining the uterus, or both are not ready for implantation. In the human, there is no evidence of death of the ovum after implantation. Whether eggs are fertilized in the presence of an IUCD is not yet known, although the devices do not prevent sperm from reaching the tubes. The hypermotility postulated in the monkey may or may not occur in man. Some Swedish workers have shown that the insertion of a loop provokes the uterus into prelabor contractions at the time when a fertilized ovum might be seeking implantation. They suggest that the IUCD's therefore disturb or prevent implantation. Some have worried that the ability to prevent a fertilized egg from implanting is not contraception but abortion. Dr. A. S. Parkes of the Physiological Laboratory at Cambridge has commented: ". . . with the . . . IUCD it is not known in any particular cycle whether an egg has been fertilized or not, because the menstrual rhythm is not disturbed. . . . I do not think you can abort a hypothetical embryo." While the argument that "what you don't know won't hurt you" will not please everyone, Parkes's attitude of moral comfort represents the majority view.

The most effective devices are probably almost as good as the pills in preventing conception. A few women expel the devices without knowing it, and thus become pregnant. A rare patient becomes pregnant while the IUCD is still in place, but this has usually not produced obstetric difficulties for either the fetus or mother. Other women have to have the devices removed for excessive or irregular bleeding, abdominal cramps, or backache. Occasionally women request removal because of lack of confidence in the technique, fear of cancer, religious scruples, or because their husbands object to the device. Those women who have early discomfort usually have no further symptoms if they can stick it out for a few months. If expulsion does not occur during the first three months of use (it usually takes place during the menses) the chances of later expulsion are low. The presence of the IUCD in the uterus may be more easily detected in the future by devices that monitor such presence from the outside, such as the deflection of a compass needle (held over the lower abdomen) by a small piece of magnetized iron incorporated into the IUCD. One Danish company makes a "Beolocator" employing a metal probe that produces a click over a loudspeaker if it touches the device. Such testing is said to take less than a minute and to be painless.

How often pelvic inflammation is caused by IUCD's is not known with precision, because such inflammation can occur in the absence of IUCD's. The incidence of such disease has been lowest with the steel ring and highest with the spiral, but this may only reflect the fact that in the early experience with these, the ring has been most used in private patients while the spiral has primarily been tried in clinic patients, who more commonly develop inflammation. Pelvic inflammation seems to respond to antibiotics whether the device is left in place or removed.

A potentially serious complication is uterine perforation. Most perforations have not been associated with serious consequences, and some devices that have passed through the uterine wall have merely been left in the peritoneal cavity. A few, however, have caused intestinal obstruction and required emergency operations. It has been proposed that most of these perforations are due to overforceful introduction or removal of the devices, or the presence of severe flexion deformities of the uterus, narrowing of the cervical opening, recent pregnancy, or uterine fibroids. The rate of perforation falls from 35 per 1,000 when done two to five weeks after confinement to 2 per 1,000 when accomplished thirteen or more weeks after confinement, and is also inversely related to the skill and experience of the fitting physician. Some devices also seem to cause more technical difficulties than others. (So far the loop looks best.) These troubles, while rare, can be important, and represent the major argument against widespread use of the IUCD's in a population that has other techniques available.[1]

Whether IUCD's may cause cancer of the uterus is not known, but to date there is no evidence that this is occurring. Nor is there reason as yet to worry that women will not be able to conceive after removal of the devices.

The biggest appeal of the IUCD's is their convenience. Once in, they can be left undisturbed for long periods. There is no sustained motivation required on the part of either sexual partner. This fact, plus the trivial expense involved, make IUCD's particularly attractive for any group unaccustomed to the contraceptive way of life.

In the past, birth control was always highly correlated with the literacy rate of a nation. Reduction of birth rate depended less on new methods than on the application of traditional

---

[1] The other main drawback to IUCD's is that they are generally unsuited to use in women who have never been pregnant.

methods after people recognized the desirability of limiting family size. The oral contraceptives were perhaps the first exception to this general rule, and they have been popular even in socio-economically benighted areas, but the IUCD's represent perhaps the ultimate in simplicity. (As one expert pointed out, if illiterate women are to control their reproduction with oral contraceptive intake timed by counting beads, they must first learn to count.)

In India, the first IUCD factory was opened in 1965. Guests at the dedication ceremony received gold-plated loops for souvenirs. The factory eventually intends to produce 14,000 plastic loops a day, an annual total of 5,000,000. In South Korea, 350,000 IUCD's had been fitted by 1966. Taiwan aims to have 600,000 fitted by the end of 1968. Other programs are under way in Tunisia, Egypt, Chile, Puerto Rico, Jamaica, Barbados, Turkey, Mexico, Hong Kong, Thailand, and more than fifty other countries.

The introduction of this technique to the United States has not been free of unsavory aspects. A loop can be made for a few pennies, and an inserter good for twenty loops for about half a dollar. Yet individual loops sell for one to two dollars, and some gynecologists charge as much as $400 for an insertion. The American College of Obstetricians and Gynecologists, via its Executive Board, has suggested that the fee should not be more than $25.

More troublesome is the Food and Drug Administration's lack of authority to regulate such devices. Since the IUCD's are not drugs, they have not been subjected to legal requirements and governmental review before marketing. Anyone who wants to sell an IUCD of any shape, size, or material can do so, without evidence of its reliability as a contraceptive or of its safety. The present laws probably require amending before the FDA can provide consumer protection in this area or in such unrelated areas as the sale of diagnostic and therapeutic machines, or prosthetic devices such as artificial limbs.

While IUCD's represent the present epitome of simple,

reversible birth control, there is another simple and effective approach to contraception that is much older—surgical sterilization. It was originally used to protect women whose life or health was threatened by pregnancy. Dr. James Blundell proposed the procedure in 1823, but it required the aseptic surgery and anesthesia of the latter part of the nineteenth century to make surgical sterilization practical. At this time, sterilizing operations on the male began to be performed, but mainly as incidental steps in connection with operations on the prostate.

With increasing confidence in its efficacy and safety, there was increased use of surgical sterilization to prevent persons with certain disorders, such as mental deficiency, psychosis, or epilepsy, from having offspring. Between 1907 and 1937, thirty-two states in this country adopted legislation regulating eugenic sterilization. Some of these laws have since been declared unconstitutional, but most are still in force, if not very often applied.

In recent years, the emphasis has been on voluntary sterilization as a birth-control measure for the general population. Vasectomy in the male is simple, does not require hospitalization, and can be done under local anesthesia. Tying a woman's tubes requires an abdominal incision, but if done right after delivery hardly lengthens the period of bed rest. These procedures are not perfect—perhaps 0.5 per cent fail to prevent conception—but they are effective, entail little risk, and are highly satisfactory for many couples. The major drawback is that a patient may come to regret the irreversibility of the act because the marriage is (or becomes) an unhappy one or because he or she had reluctantly consented after urging by the spouse. Periodically, some surgeon reports a "brilliantly successful" new operation for reopening the tubes of the female or the vasa of the male, but these usually turn out to be less satisfactory after more sober appraisal. In general, it must be assumed that a properly done sterilization is not easily reversible.

Except for the states of Connecticut and Utah, where

medical necessity is required as a justification for voluntary sterilization, there is no apparent legal bar to the procedure in the United States. It has been estimated that more than 100,-000 Americans are operated on each year, mostly people who have completed their families. Hospitals usually make up their own rules as to who is eligible; in general a young woman, or one with fewer than five children, is refused this type of surgery.

Before the pill and IUCD's, surgical sterilization was extremely popular in Puerto Rico, where perhaps 3,000 to 4,000 women were operated on yearly, in Japan, where 800,000 couples have been sterilized, and in India, where 400,000 sterilizations have been performed.

Research continues on other ways to prevent conception. One theoretical possibility is to use drugs that arrest the early development of the ovum. Another is to halt the formation of sperm. Dr. Harold Jackson of Manchester, England, has reported that chemicals are available that when given orally to male rats can render them temporarily sterile. His group hopes to develop a compound that will be safe for man and provide immediate but reversible sterility. There is a science of "immuno-reproduction" dating back to Elie Metchnikoff's 1902 publication, which aims at producing male or female antibodies to the reproductive cells themselves. By injecting an appropriate homogenate of sperm or testicular tissue into the male guinea pig, he can be made temporarily infertile. (The female guinea pig and ovary are apparently not as susceptible to such manipulation.) The theory has been that the male guinea pig develops antibodies to his own sperm, but recently it has been suggested by a Harvard researcher that the injections really provoke a disease in the pigs, rather than antibodies. Right or no, the theory is as fascinating as it is distant from clinical application.

Barely touched as yet by science is the purposeful manipulation of cultural attitudes to facilitate birth control. The small-family ideal is crucial to a successful national birth-control policy. Yet the average number of children desired by a married couple is highest in just those countries that most need population control. The average desired family is less than three in all European countries except Italy, Norway, and the Netherlands. Among the developing countries, by contrast, more than half the people typically want four or more children, and in Pakistan and Korea more than two thirds of the population say they want at least four. To date there is little to suggest success in influencing people to want small families. Even in western Europe and American countries, families claim to desire more children than they actually end up having. There is an apparent urge to have more children as one's socio-economic lot improves.

Judith Blake has suggested that the way to improve this state of affairs is to lessen the involvement of people in familial roles. She points out that the employment of women outside the home encourages the desire for small families. The difference in family size between American wives who have had no work experience and those having five years or more of work experience is one child—a difference as great as that between Catholics and non-Catholics. Female employment could affect population growth not only by its impact on desired family size, but by delaying marriage and childbearing. A policy aimed at increasing female non-home employment does not entail expense so much as the abolition of legal restrictions and cultural barriers. It is depressing to note that a country like India discourages the employment of females, and that there was a drop in the proportion of Indian working women during the first half of this century.

The role of the doctor in birth control is a complex one. Some physicians have pioneered in population-control movements, while others have vigorously opposed them. One important variable in determining doctor attitudes has been religion. Although 75 to 90 per cent of the patients of non-Catholic doctors use diaphragms or condoms, only one third of the patients of Catholic doctors do so. These differences are in part attributable to the tendency of Catholic patients to use Catholic doctors, but this is far from the whole story. A majority of Catholic doctors refuse outright the request of Catholic patients for contraceptive devices, but they are only slightly more likely to prescribe such devices for a non-Catholic patient. If the patient's reason for desiring contraception is cardiac disease or something similar rather than merely a personal preference for a small family, this may affect the decision of a Catholic doctor, but there is all too often a conflict between science and religious conscience, with the patient caught in between.

The medical profession has been slow to prepare itself for leadership in birth control. The National Academy of Sciences–National Research Council Committee on Population said in 1965 that most physicians are still not getting adequate preparation during medical school to play an effective part. Medical-school curricula are notoriously erratic in the teaching of basic reproductive physiology and anatomy, and in Canada schools teaching fertility regulation are technically in violation of the Criminal Code. Problems of maternal and perinatal mortality, abortion, sterilization, contraception, and the principles of population change are often poorly covered. A recent survey of thirty-eight obstetrics and gynecology texts found the subject of fertility regulation omitted in two thirds of them. The psychology of birth control needs more emphasis. Sex and the marriage bed involve more irrationality and taboos than most other areas of human activity, and an approach to family planning that fails to consider the emotional aspects is doomed to failure. Malthus had two basic postulates: "First, that food is necessary to the existence of man. Secondly, that the passion between the sexes is necessary and will remain nearly in its present state." There has been much debate over his conclusions, but the wisdom of his postulates is unchallenged.

There is evidence that the frozen attitude of the American medical profession on birth control is beginning to thaw. In 1937 the AMA refused to be anything but neutral on birth control, but in 1965 its Committee on Human Reproduction

issued a forthright report, asserting that recognition of the
need for population control is a matter of responsible medical
practice and that the profession could not shirk its responsibility to provide counsel and guidance.

Current concerns over population growth seem paradoxical in view of past national and scientific efforts at increasing
fertility. Most historical population policies have encouraged
more and earlier marriages and pregnancies. Augustus encouraged senators in ancient Rome to reproduce their kind, and
Colbert did the same for the French nobility and bourgeoisie,
but in most times and countries fertility has been promoted for
all socio-economic levels. Before this century, only in some
German states in the nineteenth century was there a serious
attempt to reduce population growth, with permission to marry
restricted to couples able to support a family.

Pronatalist policies have usually been of dubious efficacy.
Colbert's pensions for families with ten or more living legitimate children—at a time when infant and adult mortality rates
were high—prompted Montesquieu to describe such provisions
as aimed at the encouragement of prodigies. French legislation
between the two world wars attempted to restrict the spread of
birth control (except for the use of the condom) but could
hardly have had effect on coitus interruptus, a popular technique among the French. Even the most recent, comprehensive population policies in Belgium and Sweden have not been
convincingly shown to work. The only thing that is clear is that
a nation can look upon world population problems with a different set of spectacles than those used for scrutinizing its own.
Even within a given country, feelings can shift dramatically:
the Japanese were until recently concerned about overcrowding
their islands, but now one finds Japanese commentary expressing apprehension about excessive population control and the
ultimate disappearance of the nation in four or five centuries if
the current trend is not reversed.

In our own and other countries, research on fertility drugs
is pursued, with the intention of helping childless couples to

bear offspring. Synthetic chemicals as well as human secretions have been successfully used to induce ovulation and pregnancy. The urine of menopausal women has been a source of gonado-tropin, a pituitary hormone that stimulates the ovary. This hormone, as well as an estrogen-like chemical named clomi-phene, has in fact been too successful in some cases, with a higher than expected incidence of multiple births, including quintuplets.

The specter of atomic war has revived interest in sperm banks, so as to allow insemination of female survivors of nu-clear holocaust. Human semen has been successfully stored for prolonged periods by freezing it in liquid nitrogen. Of the women successfully impregnated with thawed semen, some have aborted but others have borne normal-term infants. The technique has applicability not solely in times of disaster but also for women whose husbands have low sperm counts or who for any reason wish to maximize the chances of fertilization by pooling semen collected at different times.

Despite the fertility needs of some individuals, the world as a whole continues to be faced with an acute population crisis, and it remains to be seen how well we can react to it. One American expert has envisioned a time when birth-control chemicals will be put into all food and water, so as to ensure the "democratic" exposure of the entire population to the same restrictions. Then an antidote would be given to those who wish to have children. It needs little imagination to concep-tualize the Orwellian horrors that are possible in such a situa-tion, and it is to be fervently hoped that man can forestall the need for nonvoluntary population control. History suggests, however, that human foresight is limited, and that the notion of cure has been more popular than the ideal of prevention. The methods for avoiding disaster are usually more obvious than the desire of man to utilize them. For population control, as for the horrors of war, the odds favor the pessimistic bettor.

9

Abortion:
Crime or Civil Right?

THERE ARE few things about which American society is more hypocritical than abortion. Although a frequently recurring estimate—which may be too high by a factor of five or ten, according to some, and too low by a few hundred thousand, according to others—is that a million U.S. pregnancies a year end in illegal abortion, the problem receives scant attention from society. As Dr. Mary S. Calderone, medical director of Planned Parenthood–World Population, has said: "The problem is not even recognized and yet any health officer worth his salt . . . would spring to panicky action if even a tiny proportion [of such numbers] of cases of any other illness appeared in his daily work."

Our laws profess a tender concern for the pregnant mother but drive her to the perils of self-induced abortion or the inadequate facilities of the criminal abortionist, conveniently overlooking the fact that the risk of dying from unwanted pregnancy is several times greater than the risk of dying from a competently performed abortion in the first three months of pregnancy.

The public continues to visualize the woman seeking abortion largely as the unwed schoolgirl or the promiscuous sexpot, ignoring the evidence that the older married woman—often with several children—is more typical. Clark Vincent, chief of the social-sciences section of the National Institute of Mental Health, has pointed out that the rate of illegitimate pregnancies has increased most, during the last two decades for which figures are available (1939–59), in women in the third decade of life. Illegitimate births rose from 9 to 37 per 1,000 live births for the twenty to twenty-four-year-old group, and 5 to 26 per 1,000 for the twenty-five to twenty-nine-year-olds, while the rate for girls under twenty has actually declined since 1938.

Legal strictures are equally hypocritical. Criminal abortion is a felony, but the mother is never, and the abortionist rarely, prosecuted. Doctors share in the hypocrisy. The majority do not perform abortions, but many are willing to recommend someone who will. The practice of therapeutic abortions in many hospitals is a medical burlesque. Most such operations are clearly unsanctioned by the law, but no one is arrested. The psychiatric indications that are now the prime reasons for therapeutic abortion are found in direct proportion to the personal enthusiasm of the doctor for liberal abortion policies.

Dr. Kenneth R. Niswander has compiled a revealing set of statistics for the city of Buffalo, New York. In two teaching hospitals there he found the incidence of therapeutic abortion among clinic patients almost equal to the incidence among private patients for the years 1943 to 1949. By the years 1960 to 1964, the incidence of therapeutic abortion among private patients had almost doubled while there was a precipitous drop among clinic patients. Nor was this the only difference: 75 per cent of the private patients who were aborted had psychiatric indications during a period when only one clinic patient was aborted for any reason—epilepsy. "Are we to conclude," asks Dr. Niswander, "that our clinic patients are emotionally more stable than those in private practice?"

In New York City the percentage of therapeutic abortions among white women is five times that among nonwhites, and twenty-six times that for Puerto Ricans. The rate of therapeutic abortions in proprietary hospitals is six times that for general-service patients in voluntary hospitals, and forty times the rate in municipal hospitals. Thus of 875 therapeutic abortions in New York City in a recent three-year period, only sixteen were performed in all of the municipal hospitals.

The trend is clearly down for total number of therapeutic abortions, while the puerperal death rate from abortion has risen. Such mortality is highest in just those women who do not readily obtain therapeutic abortions—the nonwhites and Puerto Ricans. Almost half the maternal deaths in New York City are due to criminal abortions, and the figures from California are not dissimilar. The California data show why such deaths are to be expected. The methods used to induce abortion—often by the woman herself—include injecting soap or peroxide; inserting coat hangers, knitting needles, or welding wire into the uterus; inserting air with a football pump and a straw; douching with lysol, soap, or potassium permanganate; and ingesting such things as turpentine. The toll from bloodstream infection, kidney failure, liver damage, and peritonitis is predictably high.

In the United States, the laws of most states stipulate a threat to the life of the pregnant woman as the sole legal ground on which pregnancy can be interrupted. In a few states this is extended to cases where there is any serious threat to the health of the mother. In some, there is no statutory exception to the crime of abortion.

Other countries have more liberal policies. In Sweden and Denmark, comprehensive legislation was enacted in the late 1930's, and then amended during the next two decades. In each country, the law recognizes that abortion can be performed not only for medical but for eugenic and humanitarian reasons as well Thus a woman may have her pregnancy interrupted if her "mental strength will be seriously reduced by the birth and care of her child." In recent years, 70 to 85 per cent of legal abortions in Denmark and Sweden have been performed on psychiatric grounds, including conditions described as "exhaustion."

The Swedish law of 1946 mentions only hereditary transmission of mental illness, mental deficiency, and other severe illness or defects as eugenic indications, but in fact the Royal Medical Board has authorized the interruption of pregnancy in many cases of German measles and at least one famous case of thalidomide toxicity (the American Mrs. Finkbine). Denmark also recognizes such humanitarian indications as pregnancy resulting from rape or incest or occurring in children under fifteen years of age.

The effect of the legislation was dramatic. Legal abortions in Sweden rose from about 400 in 1939 to more than 6,300 in 1951, with similar figures for Denmark. More recently, this trend has been reversed so that each country now has about 3,000 to 4,000 legal abortions per year. The reasons for this reversal are not clear. One possibility is that attitudes of pregnant women toward abortion have changed. Another is the more general and skillful use of contraceptives, including the new oral drugs.

Still another possibility is the greater use of extralegal abortion. The availability of legal abortions does not necessarily eliminate the criminal abortionist. For one thing, privacy is still prized highly by many women desiring abortion. In Sweden, there is public dissatisfaction with the medical review boards; red tape and delays cause frustration and anxiety, and a board may finally refuse to abort anyway. Women have begun to go to nearby Poland for their abortions, although they are theoretically punishable by law for such practice, as is anyone who assists in such interruption of pregnancy. Those who have facilitated contact between pregnant Swedish women and Polish obstetricians argue that the alternative for many of these women is a criminal abortion with inferior medical facilities.

Meanwhile, the Polish embassy and travel agencies in Stockholm are doing a booming business in travel visas and plane reservations for hurried, off-season vacations in Poland.

In Japan, the 1948 Eugenic Protection Law authorized interruption of pregnancy for economic as well as medical reasons. The actual interpretation of this law by all parties concerned has been such as to make abortion available practically on request. The official figures show a rise in legal abortions from 246,000 in 1949 to 1,170,000 in 1965, but the numbers are thought to be far short of the truth because of the reluctance of Japanese physicians to pay income tax on their full earnings.

In 1920, the USSR legalized interruption of pregnancy at the request of the pregnant woman. Sixteen years later a decree restricted legal abortion to a specified list of medical and eugenic indications, but in 1955 the restrictive decree was repealed. Most of the countries of eastern Europe have followed Russia's lead. The goals of legislation—at least as stated officially by the USSR—are to limit the harm from illegal abortion and to give women the right to determine motherhood for themselves. This is especially interesting since Marxist philosophy proscribes official concern with rapid population growth. At least two Communist countries—Czechoslovakia and Hungary—encourage procreation by granting family allowances for children beyond the second. As Ritchie Calder wrote in the *New Scientist:*

> It was Malthus the social reactionary who infuriated radicals from Cobbett to Marx. Karl Marx rejected the whole concept of overpopulation; the evils which Malthus was stressing were merely the results of maldistribution under capitalism and could be removed by Socialist planning. This, ignoring the legitimate demographic factors which Malthus had raised, has put dogmatic Communism alongside dogmatic Catholicism in opposition to population control.

Throughout eastern Europe, where abortion is legal, it is prohibited in pregnanices of over three months' duration except for medical reasons and is forbidden if the applicant has had an abortion during the preceding six months. Abortions for medical reasons are free, but those on request or for social indications must be paid for. The result of these laws has been a spectacular increase in legal abortions. No statistics are available for Russia, but in Hungary the number rose from 1,600 in 1949 to 170,000 in 1961, a year in which there were only 130,000 live births. In Czechoslovakia the number of legal abortions rose from 35,000 in 1955 to 120,000 in 1961. Since then it has hovered around the 100,000 mark, Czech authorities having decided in 1963 that the abortion rate was too high. In each country in eastern Europe where abortion has been legalized, there has been a decline in birth rate. In 1962, the decline ranged from 15 per cent in the USSR to 40 per cent in Hungary. No such decline was seen in Albania or East Germany, where abortion has not been legalized.

How dangerous is such readily available legal abortion? Data from Japan are strangely lacking, but the morbidity and mortality figures from eastern Europe are almost unbelievably low. There the annual death rate from legal abortion is said to range from 0 to 6 per 100,000. It is thought that this low rate reflects the restriction of most abortions to the first three months of pregnancy. In Scandinavia, for example, where this is not the case, the figures are substantially higher. There is apparently no special problem with post-abortion sterility, since the available data show an incidence of involuntary sterility that corresponds to that after obstetrical confinement.

Experts from all over the world seem unanimous in the opinion that abortion—legal and illegal—remains today the single most important method of family limitation. In Chile, for example, there are an estimated 130,000 abortions yearly compared with 290,000 live births. Of these 130,000, two thirds are criminally induced and account for most of the post-abortion complications, which occupy one quarter of the maternity beds in the National Health Service Hospitals. In

Paris there are said to be forty abortions for every hundred live births.

Uruguay, whose 1.3 per cent annual population growth rate is one of the lowest in the world, claims 150,000 abortions yearly, 80 per cent being on married women. In Guatemala, where there is also widespread use of abortion, most of the illicit procedures occur among the lower economic classes. Because these abortions are accomplished by crude methods applied by untrained people without antiseptic techniques, 15 per cent of them end in death for the mother. In Honduras, there are 17.5 per cent more abortions than live births. It is easy to see, from these various figures, why some world population experts place the total number of yearly abortions at 30,000,000—one of of every five pregnancies.

There is agitation in several countries for legal reforms that would liberalize the indications for abortion. Britain, where it has been estimated that there are somewhere between 50,000 and 250,000 criminal abortions yearly, is one such nation. Lord Silkin introduced a bill in 1966 which proposed substantial changes in British law. One provision added risk of injury, either mental or physical, to the pregnant woman as grounds for termination. Another subsection provided for abortion if there were "substantial risk that if the child were born it would suffer from such physical or mental abnormalities as to deprive it of any prospect of reasonable enjoyment of life." Still other portions of the bill allowed for termination of pregnancy if a girl was less than sixteen years of age, or if the potential mother were mentally defective. After the British Medical Association offered some constructive comments on Silkin's bill, a slightly different bill was presented to the House of Commons. After a series of amendments were added by the House of Lords to the version submitted by the House of Commons, the bill finally received the Royal Assent on October 27, 1967. The bill was expected to come into force six months or so later.

In the United States, too, there is pressure for legal reform. In 1964 the Association for Humane Abortion was founded in New York, its name being changed later to the Association for the Study of Abortion. It proposes to evaluate the attitudes of lay and professional groups toward existing abortion practices, and to assess their effect on both the individual and society as a whole. The organization is also dedicated to the education of the public regarding all aspects of the abortion problem, in the hope of achieving legal reforms through public meetings and the use of mass media.

The Society for Humane Abortion, headquartered in San Francisco, has a simple principle: "By legislating abortion, the concept remains that abortion, in itself, is wrong." The society asks, "Do you ever speak of a legal tooth extraction or a legal hysterectomy or tonsillectomy? Obviously not. Then why a 'legal' abortion?" It considers mistaken the concept that abortion is, per se, evil. Rather, "abortion is simply a surgical procedure. Surgical procedures are already protected by the health and safety code and the business and professions code. We believe that EVERY woman seeking an abortion is entitled to proper medical care."

This society actively campaigned to repeal sections 274, 275, and 276 of the California Penal Code, which made it a crime to perform an abortion except to save a woman's life. Enacted in 1872, the law was at variance with the facts of life: Most non-Catholic hospitals in the state broke the law, for example, in aborting women who contracted German measles during the first trimester of pregnancy, forty-six such cases having been aborted in 1965 at the San Francisco University of California Medical Center alone.

In several successive sessions, a Humane Abortion Act was introduced by Assemblyman Anthony Beilenson of Beverly Hills, to permit a therapeutic abortion in a hospital, on approval of a committee of the hospital, for patients who seek it when continuance of pregnancy would gravely impair the physical or mental health of the mother, or there was substantial risk of a defective child being born, or the pregnancy resulted from rape or incest.

Such reform has had backing from many individuals and groups. In 1960 and 1962, Los Angeles grand juries recommended broadened grounds for abortion. The California Medical Association, the California State Department of Health, and the leading obstetrical and gynecologic societies in California all urged reform. More than 1,000 specialists in obstetrics, pediatrics, psychiatry, and preventive medicine petitioned the California legislature in 1965 in support of the Beilenson Bill. Two hundred leading California lawyers called for enactment of the legislation. Over 1,000 clergymen of almost all denominations from 344 California cities and towns endorsed a similar resolution.

Despite strong opposition from the Catholic Church, the Assembly Committee on Criminal Procedure voted to report the bill out of committee at the end of the 1965 legislative session. Further action was prevented by weakening amendments made in committee and by adjournment of the legislature, but the bill was reintroduced and passed into law in June 1967.

Certain medical leaders have been opposed to such changes. Dr. James V. McNulty, a prominent Catholic and a member of the State Board of Medical Examiners, called the Beilenson Bill "poorly conceived, and difficult to execute." He envisions the danger of new twenty-five-bed "hospitals" which would really be abortion mills. He also apparently doesn't trust his fellow physicians: "What about the problem of collusion? . . . Should not the therapeutic abortion committee have a lay member as a safeguard against conspiracy on the part of the doctors?" Furthermore, since Dr. McNulty considers the fertilized egg not a "protoplasmic blob" but a person,[1] he points out that the bill denies to the unborn child "the right to counsel, the right to notice, the right to present evidence for his side."

In April 1966, McNulty revealed that the Board of Examiners had requested the Attorney General of California to prosecute doctors who performed abortions in cases where the life of the mother was not in danger. Apparently failing to evoke a response, the board went ahead on its own late the next month, filing disciplinary charges against two prominent San Francisco doctors who allegedly had performed hospital abortions on pregnant women who had contracted German measles. If found guilty, the doctors face possible revocation of their license to practice medicine in the state. Meanwhile, anesthetists, obstetricians, and hospitals were for a time refusing to abort such women for fear of legal action. Thus the shady criminal-abortionist business was given a lift in sunny California. The new 1967 abortion law will, it is hoped, make things easier for the conscientious doctor.

Also in New York State a fight is being waged to update antiquated laws. A leader is Dr. Robert E. Hall, a soft-spoken but hard-hitting critic of legal inadequacies. At his own Sloane Hospital for Women in New York City, Dr. Hall found one abortion per 55 deliveries among private patients, as against one in 224 ward deliveries. Abortions for psychiatric reasons occurred once in every 104 private deliveries, but only once in 1,149 ward deliveries. His poll of sixty randomly selected major hospitals in twenty-nine states and the District of Columbia showed similar trends, with abortions about four times as frequent on the private service as on the wards. As Professor R. A. Kimbrough, Jr., of the University of Pennsylvania put it: "We are aware of the tremendous disproportion. . . . It is an ugly reflection on something; I am afraid a reflection on us."

---

[1] One is reminded of the American theologian Jonathan Edwards, who outdid Calvin by damning not only infants but embryos. He declared that the floor of hell was carpeted with these poor little creatures, "some of them not even a span in length." William Pepperel Montague called this an all-time low in theological sadism.

Hall has lamented: "The American doctor is forced to practice hypocrisy.... Our laws ... force the physician to make the choice between ... good medicine and compliance with the law ... doctors should not be asked to determine which women qualify for abortions. We are no more qualified to do so than accountants or streetcleaners." Hall's position is that in the great majority of cases, health is not the issue, and that no one is better suited to decide the matter than the prospective parents.

The New York Academy of Medicine and the New York County Medical Society have proposed changes in the New York State Penal Code to recognize the health of mother and child as indications for abortion, and bills providing such changes have been placed before the New York State Assembly and Senate.

Colorado and North Carolina passed new abortion laws within a month of each other in the spring of 1967. Both were patterned after the American Law Institute's model penal code. In both states, individual doctors worked with vigor to get the controversial legislation changed. By the beginning of 1968 many of the remaining states were considering similar legislation.

The AMA has been predictably slow in its official actions. In 1965 its Committee on Human Reproduction urged the AMA to go on record as favoring uniform state laws providing that a licensed physician could terminate pregnancy if he could reasonably establish substantial risk to the physical or mental health of the mother, or risk of a defective fetus, or of pregnancy resulting from statutory or forcible rape or incest. But the House of Delegates, without discussion or an audible voice of dissent, pronounced it "not appropriate at this time ... to recommend the enactment of legislation in this manner for all states." In 1967, however, the AMA finally changed its ninety-six-year-old policy on therapeutic abortion as suggested two years earlier but did not urge uniform changes in state laws.

Meanwhile, the patients continued to search for answers to their problems. As Dr. Kenneth R. Niswander has written:

> Nearly every physician encounters a patient for whom pregnancy is a difficult social problem—whether it is a girl of 12 made pregnant by her older brother of 16, or a constantly tired and nervous woman of 40 who presents herself totally distraught at the discovery of a new pregnancy when she already has five children and an unreliable husband, financially and emotionally: she weeps, her face is drawn and horrified, and the physician realizes that he has no lawful means of helping her. Or it is a 38-year-old divorcee who is supporting three teenagers and who is pregnant by an unhappily married man unable to obtain a divorce. The wages of sin are one thing, but the injury to the teenaged children is another, and no law holds out relief. Even the physician who is bound by his beliefs to accept no indication for abortion may wish, when he is faced with one of these patients, that he could make an exception.

What other solutions have been offered to the woman who is pregnant but doesn't want to be? One is forced marriage, a dubious solution at best, and a meaningless suggestion for the majority of candidates for abortion, who are already married. A second solution is to utilize the devices of adoption, foster homes, and orphanage care. The psychiatrist Harold Rosen has responded to this proposition:

> No one has stressed . . . the heartlessness, the cruelty, and the sadism that the pregnant woman senses . . . when physician, minister, or lawyer suggests to her that she carry the child to term and then hand it over, never to see it again, to someone else to raise. Thirty-seven of the last 44 unwillingly pregnant patients referred here for consultation had, before their referral, adamantly rejected all pressure in this direction . . .
>
> During the past 18 years [I have] seen only three patients for whom "farming out" of a child for adoption would not have been exceedingly traumatic and psychiatrically contraindicated. . . . A woman does not lightly leave a baby in a basket on someone else's doorstep, or in a hospital nursery.

What is often forgotten is the undesirable disregard for the law that is encouraged by nonenforcement of the Penal Code. F. J. Taussig has written that he knew "of no other instance in history in which there has been such frank and universal disregard for criminal law." And Lord Devlin is quoted in a 1963 British report as saying: " . . . in matters of morality about which the community as a whole is not deeply imbued with a sense of sin, the law sags under a weight which it is not constructed to bear."

The legal approach to abortion attempts to cover under one umbrella a host of problems—medical, legal, ethical, and religious. Historically, the present U.S. laws reflect a concern for philosophical discussions as to the sanctity of human life, and the time at which a person becomes a person. A survey of the pronouncements of Plato, Aristotle, the Stoics, the Talmud, or Roman Catholic authorities, however, reveals that such discussions are marked by the difficulties inherent in a question that is susceptible to opinion but not proof.

Aristotle decreed that life did not begin until "quickening"—when the mother felt life in the uterus. He suggested—without biological grounds—that this happened after forty days for males and after eighty days for females. (I don't know how one was supposed to know what the sex of the young fetus was.) This rule was preserved in the sixth-century Justinian Code and dominated European abortion laws until the nineteenth century. Even the Catholic Church maintained the rule from 1244 to 1869, at which time all abortions were prohibited by the Church. In Anglo-Saxon law, abortion was not a criminal offense but an ecclesiastical one until George III's time, and even after that the quickening rule was respected. It was not until after 1861 that English law (and ultimately American) prohibited abortion at any time.

Catholic Canon Law now looks upon any attack on the unborn as a form of murder, and a violation of the commandment "Thou shalt not kill," which has been no obstacle to modern Church approval of killing in self-defense or wartime, or the practice of capital punishment. The Church draws the line at abortion as the killing of "innocent life."

Some Catholic obstetricians find difficulties even in considering the possibility of therapeutic abortion to save the life of the mother. As Dr. André Hellegers of Georgetown has asked: "How sure can I be that it was really the abortion which saved the maternal life? Will the mother die in spite of the abortion? How long will I prolong her life by the abortion? By a year? By a month? By a day?"

What society is achieving at present with its pseudo-puritanical legal strictures is death and misery for many women and their families. Garrett Hardin, professor of biology at the University of California, has aptly pointed out:

> We can force a woman to have a child. We cannot force her to want one . . . we cannot keep her rebellion from poisoning her relationship with that child, with her other children, with her husband, and indeed with society in general.
>
> . . . Critics of abortion . . . fail to realize that abortion, like other means of birth control, can lead to fulfillment. A woman who aborts this year because she is in poor health, neurotic, economically harassed, unmarried, on the verge of divorce, or immature, may well decide to have some other child five years from now—a wanted child.

And Harold Rosen has put it forcefully:

> Current abortion practices and . . . laws in the United States are incompatible with concepts of human dignity. . . . Women in our society are no longer chattel . . . as mature human beings with all the respect and dignity to be accorded mature human beings, [they] should have the right to decide whether or not they wish to carry a specific pregnancy to term. The responsibility for the decision, right or wrong, is already theirs. The extra-legal abortion rate shows that they have already illegally assumed it. It should be theirs *legally*.

10

Slaughter
of the Innocents

S OME WHO OPPOSE the use of intrauterine contraceptives do
so because they consider them instruments of murder,
believing that once a sperm and egg have united, the result is
a human being with a soul. There may be religious, philosophical, or scientific grounds for rejecting this belief, but it must
be taken into account in any consideration of the practical
application of population controls by large segments of the
world's inhabitants.

The Ortho Research Foundation of Raritan, New Jersey,
has developed a birth-control pill that might be called an
abortifacient. Known as ORF 3858, the drug is a weak estrogen
and has prevented pregnancy when given to fertile female
monkeys after mid-cycle matings. Similar contraceptive success
has been achieved with other estrogens, such as diethyl-
stilbestrol, a drug commonly taken by women to counteract
menopausal symptoms.

Such drugs have been called "after-the-fact" contraceptives. They would represent a happy alternative technique for
many women, especially those who have intercourse infre-

quently. Theoretically, at least, the side effects should be minimal compared to those of the one-a-day oral contraceptives in wide use.

After an egg has been fertilized in the Fallopian tubes, it takes up to a week or so to become attached to the uterine wall. The new Ortho pill presumably blocks implantation, and the rebuffed egg washes out of the body. In monkeys, the pill works even if taken six days after mating; preliminary data in humans with several estrogens are scanty but provide room for optimism.

The use of such a retroactive pill would be a boon to the girl who was raped or caught off guard in a moment of passion. If further experience is as encouraging as the preliminary data, medicine and society may be on the way to developing reasonably safe and effective clinical abortifacients—or at least pre-abortifacients. Other drugs, such as the antimetabolites used to treat acute leukemia, can destroy an already developing fetus, but their effects are not predictable enough unless they are given in amounts that imperil the health of the mother, and may also cause fetal deformity instead of abortion.

The religious battle lines are already forming. Although the American College of Obstetricians and Gynecologists defines life as beginning with implantation, the Catholic Dr. John Rock has said of the Ortho pill: "I wouldn't use any abortifacient any more than I would perform an instrumental abortion." (Rock presumably does not consider the possibility that the standard oral contraceptives, whose use he has so ably fostered, on occasions fail to inhibit ovulation but still work by preventing implantation. The successful experimental use of "mini-dose" progestogens, which prevent pregnancy without inhibiting ovulation, suggest that the standard oral contraceptives can work in this way.) The Protestant National Council of Churches has the question under study, and the British Council of Churches has already accepted any contraceptive that works before implantation. A. S. Parkes of Cambridge University has put it as follows: "I have repeatedly stated my view as a biologist that conception means implantation of the fertilized egg, not fertilization itself; and you cannot cause abortion before conception has taken place . . . I am prepared to argue the point with biologists, bureaucrats, bishops or any others who wish to take issue . . ."

Killing of newborn infants, although popular in ancient times in different parts of the world and practiced in modern times by some primitive tribes, is out of fashion today. Infanticide has not always been simply a matter of population control: in Madagascar, as recently as a few decades ago, all children born on certain unlucky days were allegedly put to death to prevent them from bringing bad luck to their families. Such a method of population control was presumably quite acceptable in preliterate societies where a child's life was not held sacred until he had gone through some formal ceremony of tribal recognition. Until such time, he could be killed by the parents without compunction.

It is argued that infanticide meets the needs of primitive groups more effectively than does contraception, which limits the population in an uncertain, hit-or-miss manner. Infanticide can both limit the population in relation to the food supply and control the sex ratio. Thus a hunting culture might prefer a surplus of males, an agricultural society a surplus of females.

It seems unthinkable that modern society should utilize infanticide for any purpose. But as a medical student I remember being told that it was not rare for doctors to omit orders for a sulfa drug or penicillin when a mongoloid child had pneumonia because it was kinder to let the child die. And more subtle ways exist for doctors to cut such retarded children off from life. I refer to the still all too prevalent tendency to recommend institutionalization of a mongoloid child as soon as possible after birth. The rationale is that keeping such a child at home is completely disrupting to the family. The child upsets the parents and the other children and completely monopolizes the time and energy of the mother.

As a young physician, I thought this philosophy thor-

oughly humanitarian—indeed, I was never exposed to any
other approach. Many years later, however, our seventh child
was born a mongoloid. He was atypical enough to be misdiag-
nosed as normal by both our obstetrician and a prominent expert in mental retardation, although the correct diagnosis was
promptly made by our own pediatrician.

There next followed a dreadful period of doubt during
which it became clearer and clearer that the child was retarded,
but we clutched at straws, hoping that he was not. Acceptance
of the truth was followed by a more important and useful
period of education. In retrospect, I realized how little discussion there has been, during medical school and house-staff
training, of mental retardation as a societal problem. It was
both shocking and humiliating to learn how ignorant I was
about a disorder that affects—in some degree or form—3 per
cent of our population. Most distressing of all was the painful
truth that the great variability among mongols in mental
capacity and potential trainability is not evident at birth, so
that the most capable and experienced pediatrician cannot
advise parents rationally on whether or not a child will ultimately have to be institutionalized. The automatic recommendation, therefore, to put away all mongols is as unscientific as
it is lacking in regard for the right of a deformed child to be
treated with the respect due a human being, with a human
capacity to learn and a human capacity to feel.

Mongols need love no less than other children. They
require especially individualized rearing, particularly during
the critical early years. They need stimulation and companionship. Being prone to infections, they thrive better in small
living groups. For all of these reasons, the right kind of home
environment serves the welfare of a mongoloid child far better
than most institutions.

From the standpoint of the family itself there are
very real advantages in caring for its own retarded member.
For mother and father, there is the warm satisfaction to be

derived from a parent-child relationship that works. Mongoloids are often extremely lovable children, sweet and affectionate. There is an added measure of emotion when a head resting gently and trustingly on your shoulder belongs to a child in special need of love and help. The excitement and pleasure of watching a youngster achieve certain goals is, if anything, greater when the child's rate of development is much slower than that of a normal child.

For the other children in the family the presence in the home of a retarded child can be an extraordinarily meaningful and beneficial experience. The normal siblings have an opportunity to develop real understanding for the handicapped and a feeling for the broad spectrum of individual differences and genetic endowment. A tolerance for the physiologically underprivileged is a valued acquisition at any age, and the younger it can be achieved, the better.

This is not to deny that there are disadvantages. The delayed period of infancy is inconvenient and will demand more than the usual supply of parental patience. Training and education require extra attention and careful planning. The parents of a mongoloid child will have to battle for the rights of their child in a society that as yet feels no sense of outrage at the lack of educational facilities for every handicapped person. The feelings of parent and child alike may take a beating in a world that exaggerates the importance of normalcy and physical beauty. Other members of the family will have to settle for a smaller share of the parents' time with a mongol in the family.

There is also no question that in certain situations a child with mongolism is better off in an institution than at home. An unstable mother who cannot face up to the task of rearing a retarded child and who is thrown into panic or depression by the continued responsibility will not help the child, herself, or other members of the family. But most parents should approach the decision in a spirit of hope and optimism, rather than guilt and despair.

Some mongols will be able to achieve a quasi-independent status, proudly earning wages for work well done. There are thousands of children born every year with congenital defects, many of them more incapacitating than mongolism. Thousands of other children develop or acquire crippling diseases, from multiple sclerosis to muscular dystrophy, from nephritis to rheumatic heart disease. Children show a tremendous range of talents and abilities, from the genius to the uneducable, from the star athlete to the physically crippled. We cannot institutionalize all who make life more difficult for their parents or siblings or deprive further those already penalized by nature. Instead we should help all our young to fulfill themselves, to make the most of what they have, to live lives that are as joyous and productive as we and they can make them.

What is especially frightening about society's lack of concern for the mentally retarded is the accumulating evidence that the handicapped child can be helped to lead a life far more satisfactory than was dreamed a few decades ago. The first step is acceptance of the concept that the retardate is not a subhuman monster split off from mankind, but a member of the lower end of the continuous spectrum of human ability. The enlightened leaders of society must accept the premise that the trainable and educable retardate should, wherever possible, take his place in the open community. Even the less fortunate may be able to function in sheltered workshops or engage in occupational therapy within an institution, and thus at least expand the horizons of their restricted world.

Some progress has been made because of the intense interest of the late President Kennedy and his family. They knew the problem at first hand, since the President's retarded sister has for many years been confined within an institution. In October 1961, Kennedy said: "We as a nation have for too long postponed an intensive search for solutions to the problems of the mentally retarded. That failure should be corrected." Six days later he appointed a panel to prepare a national plan. The panel offered ninety-five separate recommendations as a blueprint for action, and a number of these have been implemented. The 88th Congress, for example, passed two important bills that President Kennedy signed shortly before his assassination. These provide each state with funds for planning mental-retardation programs. Matching funds are available to provide maternal and child care to prevent retardate problems related to such perinatal factors as prematurity, infections, malnutrition, and birth injuries. There are also funds for construction and for training personnel.

The happiest way to deal with mental retardation is to prevent it. Those inborn defects that are generally considered amenable to treatment—such as phenylketonuria[1] and galactosemia—highlight our pathetic stupidity about the majority of retardates. Over three fourths of the 6,000,000 retarded in the United States have no recognizable organic cause for their deficiency. How many such cases might be prevented or alleviated by new discoveries is anyone's guess, but it takes no seer to predict that without additional research institutes and research programs devoted to mental retardation there will be little progress.

It is also obvious that we are not making optimal use of the things we already know. There is a pitiful lack of special education programs and of teachers with experience directed to the care of the retarded. There is not enough scholarly attention to the problems of the family with the retarded child—problems that are sociological, religious, and legal as well as medical.

The retardate's needs are always special. To the pediatrician, he may pose special feeding and infectious problems. To the testing psychologist, hearing and speech authority, neurologist, and psychiatrist, he will present a host of interrelated problems of diagnosis and correction of special sensory, motor, or emotional defects.

[1] The controversy over PKU is discussed in Chapter 15.

The education of the retarded is a difficult matter about which to generalize. There is perhaps agreement that the earlier the education begins, the better, but beyond that there are few rules. It is difficult to predict with any precision the optimum extent and duration of useful education. Intelligence tests are of limited help, since the defects of these children are often insular in nature—one mongol, for example, may speak at an early date but have poor motor development, whereas another will have surprisingly good neuromuscular coordination years before vocabulary begins to develop. An obvious conclusion is that a great deal of individualization will be required, with a low pupil-to-teacher ratio.

Some kinds of employment are feasible for the retarded, and it is evident that they do many jobs, especially stereotyped ones, very well. Indeed, certain monotonous tasks may be more efficiently performed by a retardate than by a more endowed worker who would become bored. The increasing use of the retarded in semiskilled or unskilled jobs in industries, homes, and hospitals—jobs that are now going begging—may provide a way to make such people taxpayers rather than tax consumers.

How poorly we are handling the problem at present may perhaps be appreciated by looking at some figures from California, a relatively enlightened state in regard to retardation. A compilation of applications to state hospitals revealed that 2,300 mentally retarded were on the waiting list. The California legislature, suitably jolted by the estimate, strongly urged the construction of a fifth 2,000-bed state hospital for the retarded.

The true situation called for quite a different approach, as an analysis of the applicants showed. Of the 2,300 cases, only 1,719 had been fully evaluated. Of these, less than 25 per cent were considered to require psychiatric hospitalization. Another 17.5 per cent needed medical or surgical hospitalization, not psychiatric institutionalization. Of the other 1,000 patients, about a quarter really required foster homes, 7 per cent needed nursing care, and a third could have been cared for at home if there were available adequate day care, attendant care, homemaker services, special education classes, parent counseling, and financial assistance.

Dr. Stafford C. Warren, Special Assistant to the President for Mental Retardation, estimated in 1964 the needs of an average American community of 100,000. In such a town, 3,000 persons suffer from some form of mental retardation. Perhaps 2,500 of these are mildly retarded, and less than 100 are severely affected. These children and adults all require diagnostic and counseling services. The mildly retarded preschool children, many of whom live in slums or in otherwise depressed circumstances, need welfare, social, and educational services. Public-health nursing and homemaker services are required to assist in caring for the moderately and severely retarded infants and young children. Forty special educational classes would accommodate the 600 mildly retarded pupils who with special training can become self-sufficient adult citizens, and twelve special educational classes could transform the 100 moderate or trainable retarded into productive workers in protective, supervised settings. The few severely retarded children unable to profit from formal schooling should have the use of a day-care recreation center. The 150 mildly retarded young adults who can become self-sufficient, independent, working members of the community require vocational counseling, job training, and placement services, and the 250 moderately retarded adults of all ages who can contribute to their own and the community's welfare if given an opportunity to work in a protected environment need sheltered workshops. The 56 severely retarded adults, who may never take their place as workers in the community but are no less important from the humanitarian and social viewpoint, should have activity centers, and residential centers must be provided to meet the needs of those of the retarded with problems of care and training so complex as to require twenty-four-hour effort.

Not a single community in the United States—or anywhere else—is meeting these requirements. We are willing to allocate billions to build atomic bombs and warplanes or to let a man walk in outer space, but we will not spend enough money to let our handicapped build useful lives or walk with dignity in this world. It is a strange kind of inhumanity that tolerates so barbarous a set of priorities, and we must all share in the shame.

The very members of our society who need the most help to take advantage of their limited native endowment are most handicapped in their attempts at fulfillment. Except for the families of retardates, the local and national associations for mental retardation, and a few scientific, political, and lay leaders, the public is blind to the needs of the handicapped— needs that are urgent and immediate, not hypothetical and distant. We may, as a society, scorn the civilizations that slaughtered their infants, but our present treatment of the retarded is in some ways more cruel.

The Control of Heredity: Dream or Nightmare?

T HE KNOWLEDGE that some forms of congenital defects and retardation are related to chromosomal abnormalities has stimulated hope that by manipulating the genetic makeup of the cell, we may be able to reverse deformities. The chemist Wendell M. Stanley, a Nobel Prize winner, has predicted that the next century will find mankind able to control the hereditary traits of living things to a remarkable degree. H. J. Muller, another Nobel Prize winner, also foresees mankind guiding its own evolution. The notion that man may be able to manipulate his genetic endowment is at once exciting and troublesome. How accurate are such predictions likely to be, and how desirable is the prospect of their fulfillment?

Man's ability to modify heredity in plants is well known and accepted: Luther Burbank with his ingenious, painstaking cross-pollination experiments produced more than the Shasta daisy and the Burbank potato—he revolutionized plant breeding. Hybrid corn and other crops are now commonplace; little of what we eat from the plant kingdom has not been affected by human selection superimposed on the more ancient and fundamental process of natural selection. Our wines are produced from genetically selected grapes combining the best aspects of French and American vines, and our bread comes from wheat strains repeatedly altered by human attempts to grow hardy and healthy plants.

Important as these genetic plant experiments have been, the unpredictable life history of new strains has pointed up a serious dilemma for those who would guide evolution. Marquis wheat, for example, was introduced because it was resistant to a cereal grain affliction picturesquely known as "stinking smut." The strain was indeed almost Comstockian in its disdain for smut, but unfortunately lacked the resistance of other varieties of wheat to another pest, known simply as "scab." Ceres wheat, another strain introduced with high hopes, at first was able to withstand "stem rust," but the rust retaliated with a new mutant of its own, to which Ceres proved pathetically susceptible.

Selective breeding is also an old story in the animal and bird kingdoms. For centuries thoroughbred horses have been specially bred for speed. Man o' War and other famous stallions have sired long lines of fast-running steeds. The American Kennel Club lists over a hundred breeds of purebred dogs, all carefully developed by man. The Rhode Island Red, a once broody species of hen, has been genetically guided over the years so that now only 2 per cent (instead of 91 per cent) of such fowl hatch their own eggs, the other 98 per cent being content to concentrate on laying, leaving mechanical incubators to finish the job, a situation somewhat analogous to the decline of breast-feeding in the human female.

As with the plant experiments, there have been sobering lessons in the field of animal genetics. Breeding for certain desirable qualities usually involves the sacrifice of other qualities. Race horses are swift but would be at a loss on a farm or pulling a wagon. Cows can provide either milk or good steaks, but not both.

In ages past, man was presumably as subject to the law of natural selection as other kinds of life. It is thought, for example, that the pigmented skin of the African Negro facilitated survival in a sunny, hot climate. With the coming of modern times, however, the law of the jungle has been drastically modified for man. Civilization now protects certain physically inferior individuals from ready extermination, although it is still powerless to affect the basic course of most defectives. The child with amaurotic idiocy, for example, still usually begins to lose his sight by seven and is dead by adolescence, victim of a "lethal gene."

Modern man, however, uses other forms of selection. Marriage is one such form. Married couples consciously or unconsciously make a genetic choice in picking a spouse. It may be based on nothing more than an apprehensive glance by the prospective groom at what the girl's mother looks like, but it is still a choice. There is also a certain amount of inbreeding due to the cohesive or divisive effects of economic level, education, religion, and even political views.

There are more scientific methods available, of course. The techniques for artificial insemination, first performed in man by the eighteenth-century English surgeon John Hunter, are well worked out, although present religious and legal restrictions drastically limit their use. Estimates on the number of successful artificial inseminations in the United States range from a few thousand to 100,000. And even these cannot be classified as novel eugenic measures; they are simply attempts to fertilize a childless wife with the sperm of a nameless donor chosen less for any unusual talents than for physical characteristics which will not betray the child's offbeat conception.

Even frozen sperm has been successfully employed for this purpose. Spermatozoa were first frozen by U. Mantegazza in

1866, and a number of normal pregnancies have resulted from sperm frozen for as little as forty-eight hours and as long as two and a half years.

Some scientists have predicted the use of more unusual techniques, including extracorporeal mating made possible by the preservation of both sperm and ova in test tubes, a sort of Pyrex gamete bank. It would still be necessary for a willing lady to serve as an incubator in which such a fertilized ovum could develop, although an artificial uterus or placenta is not out of the question. Facilities of this type conjure up a vision of long-distance adultery—in both a temporal and spatial sense—between total strangers. What if such a method had been available centuries ago? The fanciful notion of offspring derived from Albert Einstein and Queen Elizabeth I, or Linus Pauling and Madame de Staël, or Martha Graham and Thomas Jefferson has a certain awesome wonder about it, although the idea of mixing the gametes of Jack the Ripper and Florence Foster Jenkins gives one pause. (One also recalls Bernard Shaw's comment on the suggestion of a lady from Zurich with the "most beautiful body in the world" that they produce a super-baby: "What if the child inherits my body and your brains?")

Other possibilities have been described. Someday, we may be able to substitute, within a human nucleus, one chromosome or part of a chromosome for another, or perhaps manipulate a chromosomal change by purposely introducing a virus with a special affinity for the genetic markers we wish to alter. Although we can make shrewd guesses about the relationship of specific chromosomes and many bodily traits, our information is still rudimentary. There are billions of nucleotide units in each set of chromosomes, and change in any one is likely to have important (and at present unpredictable) effects. This type of manipulation—potentially the most important—is still far off in the future so far as man is concerned.

Given the availability of one or more of the approaches mentioned, however, how desirable is this meddling with heredity? Some of it has already been of considerable benefit to man. The original *Penicillium* mold was not a highly efficient penicillin producer, but irradiation provided new strains capable of substantially higher yields. The production of hardier, improved sources of vegetables, fruits, and meat has been of great importance to man.

But the evolutionary guidance of man himself is much more complex and raises questions of what goals are appropriate, who the genetic judges are to be, and whether there is to be consent on the part of the individuals at risk in any evolutionary experiments. Perhaps the least controversial area of genetic control would be the restitution of some congenitally abnormal individuals to relative normality. One of the most consistent chromosomal abnormalities is that associated with the defect of mongolism; such individuals most commonly have an extra chromosome. If a normal chromosomal complement could somehow be induced in these mongoloid children, one might thereby eliminate their physical and mental inadequacies. Few would damn such interference with nature; it would be a merciless kind of religious scruple that relentlessly demanded a full measure of mental and somatic retardation.

Chromosomal substitution of the type referred to above would also seem less objectionable than the harsh genetic quarantine applied to the Fore Tribe by the government of New Guinea. The tribe suffers from a fatal neurological disease called kuru, and the 30,000 tribesmen have been forbidden to migrate from their 884 square miles of reservation, so as to prevent intermarriage with other tribes. It is even more nightmarish when one considers that Drs. Gadjusek, Gibbs, and Alpers of the National Institute of Neurological Diseases and Blindness have data that strongly suggest that kuru is actually a virus infection. These scientists took brain tissue from victims of kuru and injected extracts of it into the brains of chimpanzees. The animals developed symptoms astonishingly similar to those of the human disease twenty to twenty-six months later.

The possibility of improving the whole human race brings us into still more troubled waters. Man is not perfect, to be sure. He tires readily, wastes too much time in sleep, learns slowly and imperfectly; is often needlessly cruel, fearful, greedy, and dishonest; communicates with difficulty even with his own species and not at all with most others; and loses his hair, teeth, and sexual drive as he gets older. Then there are all the diseases to which he is prey. When one remembers that even Egyptian mummies show evidence of arthritis, atherosclerosis, hernia, and gallstones, it seems high time for man to do something about such "modern" diseases.

But what traits are we sure that we want to breed out? If we were picking the superparents of the future, whom would we choose? Would Beethoven be ruled out because of his deafness? Wagner for his psychopathic attitudes? Dostoevski as an epileptic? Oscar Wilde and possibly Leonardo da Vinci and Michelangelo as homosexuals? Darwin himself was either a chronic invalid or a hypochondriac.

Why not get rid of the bad traits and keep the good? Did Wagner have to be amoral to write *Tristan*? Perhaps not, but one must remember the lessons of Marquis wheat and the thoroughbred horses. It is not inconceivable that one might breed out schizophrenia and breed in cancer. Even the dread sickle-cell condition, which in its full expression produces a severe disease characterized by anemia and a host of other troubles, is now thought by some experts to help its victims survive malaria in tropical climes.

It is also well to recall the dangers involved in disturbing the ecology of nature. A relatively small change in an environment that is in a state of dynamic equilibrium may wreak havoc. The starling, imported into this country in 1890 because of its insect-eating propensities, has turned out to be a thorough nuisance, crowding out more desirable birds such as thrushes, bluebirds, and woodpeckers, and soiling statues, buildings, and pedestrians with its droppings. The measles virus decimated the Faroe Islanders in 1846 when it was suddenly brought into the community from Copenhagen. One has to fear not only the possible effects of genetic novelty in the altered individuals, but the effects of such newcomers on their neighbors and on life at large.

One must also worry considerably about who is to manipulate the hereditary traits. Who shall have life-and-death power to make the difficult value judgments? The intolerance of persons in authority for dissidents, nonconformists, and malcontents is further cause for concern. Pick the appropriate moment in history and you could have obtained a governmental decree branding as genetically undesirable such dangerous radicals as Galileo, St. Joan, Gandhi, Luther, and Jesus Christ.

At the risk of being considered old-fashioned, I should like to express the hope that mankind will largely confine its genetic experiments to voluntary acts, such as spouse-choosing, and to the correction of gross congenital defects. There appears little reason for optimism concerning the ultimate wisdom of scientists or politicians in changing evolution.

Scientists cannot be expected to act in any other way but to accelerate our now limited abilities along the lines of genetic control. It is inconceivable that science could forsake the search for the riddle of existence because of the possibility that man will misuse the accumulated information. Einstein would be as shocked today as most living physicists are about the radioactive poisoning of our atmosphere and the threat of world incineration, but he—even anticipating our present troubles— would probably not have tried to destroy atomic knowledge, if only because of the certainty that scientific discovery hidden by a few will be uncovered by others in time.

One solution might be to cultivate empathy, humility, a capacity for fulfillment, and an appreciation of what C. S. Peirce called "fallibilism"—the principle that man can never attain absolute certainty concerning questions of fact. These traits will help us to deal with the problems of today as well as those of the morrow, with the problems of our neighbor as well as our own. They will help us make the most of the precious time, minds, and bodies we now own. They will remind us that even a deaf, blind child can appreciate the sweet morning fragrance of a pine forest or the smell of honeysuckle on a summer evening.

12

The Tyranny
of Senescence

I N 1905 William Osler delivered his valedictory address to
the Johns Hopkins University, a few weeks before leaving
America to assume new responsibilities as Regius Professor of
Medicine at Oxford. The title of the address was from a work
by Trollope:

> ... In that charming novel, *The Fixed Period*, Anthony
> Trollope discusses the practical advantages in modern life of
> a return to this ancient usage, and the plot hinges upon the
> admirable scheme of a college into which at sixty men retired
> for a year of contemplation before a peaceful departure by
> chloroform. ... The teacher's life should have three periods,
> study until twenty-five, investigation until forty, profession
> until sixty, at which age I would have him retired on a double
> allowance. Whether Anthony Trollope's suggestions of a
> college and chloroform should be carried out or not I have
> become a little dubious, as my own time is getting so short.

Although there is no evidence that his audience was of-
fended by the speech, the wayward press transformed Osler's
humorous remark into a serious plea for mandatory euthanasia

at sixty years of age. Abuse poured down on Osler's head. Senator William Stewart of Nevada, seventy-seven years old, said he could now understand Osler's "numerous failures" in caring for "Senator Hanna, Speaker Reed, Postmaster General Payne, and other distinguished Americans." Some critics penned sarcastic poems; cartoonists had a field day.

In Baltimore a seventy-one-year-old Confederate veteran shot and killed himself. In St. Louis a seventy-two-year-old man was found dead, an empty bottle of chloroform beside him. Both men's effects contained newspaper clippings about Osler's speech. The public, prompted by the newspapers, began to use the word "oslerize," and plans to erect an academy of medicine building bearing Osler's name were scrapped because of the withdrawal of subscriptions.

Two years later, a saddened Osler wrote:

> To one who had all his life been devoted to old men, it was not a little distressing to be placarded in a worldwide way as their sworn enemy, and to every man over sixty whose spirit I may have thus unwittingly bruised, I tender my heartfelt regrets. Let me add, however, that the discussion which followed my remarks has not changed, but has rather strengthened my belief that the real work of life is done before the fortieth year and that after the sixtieth year it would be best for the world and best for themselves if men rested from their labours.

The aged constitute an increasingly large body of citizens in the developed countries. In 1900 there were 3,000,000 people in the United States over 65; by 1985 there will be about 25,000,000. Their needs are clearly not to be denied, and it is the purpose of this chapter to examine the doctor's responsibilities to this segment of society.

First, however, it may be useful to ask what we know about the physiology of aging. Senescence can be defined as the gradual series of changes that result in a decreased capacity for survival on the part of the individual. It is by death, therefore, that aging is really measured—the increasing probability of death with increasing chronological age.

It is a common fallacy to assume that aging is inevitable, a characteristic of life itself. This does not seem to be the case, and it is necessary to consider the possibility that in fact the process we call aging is only the accumulated result of multiple assaults—recognized and occult—from the environment.

Natural death does not occur among unicellular organisms, where the individual and reproductive cells are one and the same. There are species of the protozoan paramecium as well as bacteria and yeasts that can go indefinitely, even without the invigorating pleasures of periodic sexual crossing. Some coelenterates go on living for a very long time without obvious loss of vitality. Specimens of *Sagartia troglodytes* were left for decades in a glass jar by Jessie Nelson, an English spinster. They lived from at least 1862 to the early 1940's, when they were all found mysteriously dead in the aquarium of the Department of Zoology of Edinburgh University.

Nor are the great differences only between phyla. Even within a species there is great variation in life span, with superannuated individuals in each class. Thus, a flatworm has been known to live for over thirty-five years, a beetle larva for forty-five years, an elephant for fifty-seven, a crow for sixty-nine, and turtles for as long as a century and a half. Except for the turtle, man is probably the only animal capable of living for more than a century. Part of the human superiority in life span is presumably attributable to the buffering powers of civilization: banded American robins, for example, usually survive less than two years in the wild, whereas captive robins have reached the age of 13 years.

No one knows how old the oldest man has been. The Biblical Methuselah lived an amazing, if unbelievable, 969 years. Thomas Parr, whose postmortem examination was performed by the discoverer of blood circulation, William Harvey, is said to have lived over 152 years, but there is no convincing evidence to support the claim. (It is equally unclear why the British chose to bury him in the Poet's Corner in Westminster Abbey, although perhaps the fact that Parr is said to have had an illegitimate child by Katherine Mitton when he was 102 years old suggests poetic fancy on somebody's part.)

From time to time some wizened old person emerges out of obscurity with a claim to excessive longevity, but almost invariably the vital records are unavailable to corroborate the claim. A decade ago an elderly Colombian male said to be 147 was taken to a medical center in New York City, where the most sophisticated measurements allowed the doctors to conclude that he was "certainly very old." The Colombian government, undaunted by the ambiguous results of the attempt to date the old gentleman physiologically, issued a postage stamp bearing his portrait and the old man's formula for longevity: "Don't worry, drink a lot of coffee, smoke a good cigar!" (How fortunate that the motto fit in so well with South American industrial products.)

The last reputed American Civil War veteran, Walter Washington Williams, who was buried with full military honors a month after his "117th" birthday, was later shown to have been five years old in 1860, and therefore undeserving of the monthly pensions he had received from the federal government and the state of Texas. In contrast, the Canadian papers are apparently impeccable in support of the claim that Pierre Joubert, a French-Canadian bootmaker, was the oldest man known to modern authenticated records, having died at the age of 113 years, 124 days.

According to one way of looking at the world, organisms can be said to fall into three general categories. One group never gets around to aging because its members decide to form new organisms before senescence has a chance to occur. The second category can be said not to age, because individual parts that are lost or wear out are continually replaced. The third category—into which man presumably falls—ages because reparative or retroactive processes fail or are absent. While man cannot hope to enter the first category, there seems no intrinsic reason why the second is out of his reach.

There are increasing attempts, for example, to replace the diseased human heart with nonliving pumps or with a living heart from another living donor. To those who view the heart romantically it may be unnerving to contemplate its replacement by a gadget, no matter how ingenious. Still, if "blue babies" can benefit from drastic rerouting of their great vessels, and if defective arteries and valves can be replaced with nonliving substitutes, the heart may also be expendable. And, if the vascular system can be renovated, so may other systems. Once we begin to speculate, it is an easy jump to more challenging questions: Is the human body an efficient mechanism? Would it be possible to design a better one that would both work better and last longer?

The classic approach to the evaluation of man as a machine determined efficiency from the ratio of work performed to energy spent. Investigators would put a normal man on a bicycle ergometer and calculate his efficiency at something like 20 per cent, a performance comparing not unfavorably with that of the horse (25 per cent), the steam engine (10 per cent), or the gasoline engine (20 to 30 per cent).

But appraising the effectiveness of the human body calls for more sophisticated and appropriate measures. Even muscular activity can spend energy without doing work. And there is secretory work (performed, for example, by such glands as the acid-forming cells of the stomach) that cannot really be thought of in the same terms as muscular work.

A lot of the body's energy goes into physiological holding actions. The organism must maintain its biological status quo within fairly narrow limits or suffer serious and perhaps irreversible damage. The acidity and alkalinity of the body, its temperature, its metabolism—such functions have to be finely regulated in the face of environmental vicissitudes that may be very great indeed.

The preservation of a relatively stable state of biological

equilibrium might be compared to the efforts of the legendary Dutch boy with his finger in the dike. Neither activity would get much credit in an analysis of work based on "force times distance" standards, but one doesn't need to be a tulip grower to appreciate the importance of that famous Dutch one-finger exercise. An analysis of the complex functions of individual organs of the body makes even more apparent how crude and irrelevant have been past attempts to calculate the efficiency of the human machine.

Suppose one wanted to measure the quantity of work done by the liver—where would one start? Some think of this organ as an abdominal mischief maker that exists solely for the benefit of the hepatitis virus or temperance crusades, but an awareness of the multiplicity of hepatic functions must generate respect, if not fondness, for a noble viscus. The liver makes, stores, extracts, excretes, detoxifies, is indispensable to protein, carbohydrate, and fat metabolism—in short, it performs dozens of tasks with an efficiency that makes any modern manufacturing plant look like the demented creation of a subnormal Australian bushman. Furthermore, in regard to some hepatic functions, such as protein synthesis, the liver is infinitely more efficient than any other "machine" available, since only the liver knows how to do the job.

We often hear nowadays of the magnificence of computers, but consider the miracle of miniaturization represented by the human brain. A computer that even began to approach the scope of its activities would need to be housed in a large building.

In appraising the ultimate complex reality of human output, we find ourselves still less able to determine the efficiency of the human body. For we are impaled on the horns of a dilemma: easily measured phenomena are often, of necessity, either severely restricted or trivial; for important aspects of human performance, we often lack readily available yardsticks of efficiency.

Thus one can ask how much work is required to move a

certain amount of air in and out of the chest, and for a given person, at a given time, under given conditions, the answer can be stated with modest precision and has meaning in the evaluation of pulmonary disease. One can similarly ask how much energy is expended in running the 100-yard dash, and anticipate an answer of some sort. But one cannot summarize in physical terms the grace of an Olympic champion running this distance, or talk thermodynamically of the "efficiency" of Ulanova dancing *Swan Lake* or of Shakespeare writing *Hamlet.*

Before we can talk intelligently about improving the human body, we must be sure that we understand the body we already possess, and we must be sure that we know what changes are desirable. These two levels of knowledge are closely intertwined; medical science will not come up with a "build-yourself-a-better-kidney" kit until it understands the kidney a great deal better than at present. Nor will it be sufficient to know, even in the greatest detail, the working of any one organ in isolation. For it is in the extraordinary coordination of its parts that the human body excels as a machine. Tinkering with some vital mechanism may do unpredictable damage to the entire apparatus, as Aesop recognized: "They found that even the belly, in its dull quiet way, was doing necessary work for the body, and that all must work together or the body will go to pieces."

Let us for a moment, however, pretend that we possess enough understanding of the human mechanism to ask whether it would be possible to change it in some way so as to improve its normal appearance or performance. Some would plead for bodies that are generally more beautiful and attractive than those we now possess. But the full Italian lips of Sophia Loren might represent thin-lipped asceticism to the Ubangis. The flat-chested heroines who once enlivened the cartoons of John Held, Jr., would starve in Hollywood today, just as Miss Mammary Wilshire of 1968 may in turn be the next generation's wet nurse and no more.

A TV cowboy less than six feet tall is usually a failure, but to say the same of an astronaut would be ridiculous. And if one has to survive for extended periods in central Africa on near-starvation rations, it may be best to be a pygmy.

One may also question the need to sleep away a quarter to a third of our lives. But how many people would want a twenty-four-hour day that they needed to fill with work or leisure of some kind? What would we do in place of sleep? Those who are already bored with life, unable to create or enjoy or relax, might find their existence as repellent as that of the characters in Sartre's *No Exit*. Even those happy few who now manage to live productively and joyously might not be more productive or happy with the new arrangement.

The best of our bones will break, and it would be exciting for engineers to come up with a metal substitute that is light, resilient, unbreakable, rustproof, and requires no lubrication. But bones are more than mere girders and struts. They also serve as reservoirs for salts and minerals for the rest of the body, and their marrow produces blood components without which the body would fall prey to hemorrhage, oxygen deficiency, or infection. It is therefore an extraordinarily complicated problem that the engineer must solve if he is to give us better bones.

The brain? Everyone can name dozens of people whose neurons need rewiring, even if one's own always seem reasonably satisfactory somehow. But it is not clear what sort of changes we want, or what brains we need in greater numbers. Physicists' or clowns'; biologists' or athletes'; composers' or chess players'; artists' or inventors'?

Perhaps we should focus on the emotional aspects of the brain. What affect shall we eradicate—greed, aggressiveness, hatred, bigotry, violence? Do we merely remove, or do we replace—and with what? This may not be the best of possible worlds, but it is far from the worst. We must beware lest we trade Candide for Pangloss. A life that calls for satirization is preferable to an existence that is a tragic, desperate masque glorifying ennui.

William James pointed out that in abolishing even war we should strive for a "moral equivalent," lest we attenuate those virtues generated by conflict. J. Bronowski, more recently, has emphasized man's strong need for violence and scapegoats. There must be a happy middle ground for human life somewhere between nuclear catastrophe and a perpetual prayer meeting, but the achievement of a happier world by a purposeful redesign of the human brain seems beyond even our dreams at present.

In regard to diseased tissue, however, we can surely expect progress. Even now we are able not only to bob noses, fit artificial eyes or limbs, graft skin, and drive hearts electronically with pacemakers, but to transplant kidneys from one person to another. The physician of today can boast of blood, cornea, and bone banks, and his successor in 2000 A.D. will probably render the sick whole in ways we can barely guess at today. Given sufficient time, man may eventually improve the efficiency of his normal, undiseased self. Meanwhile, he might take solace in the Old Testament words: "I am fearfully and wonderfully made."

THE HUMAN MORTALITY curve is not a simple, continuous function. At the very beginning of man's life there is an increased risk of dying, but the rate quickly drops to the very low one typical of most of infancy and childhood. Between ten and thirty years of age there is a barely perceptible increase in rate, followed by a snowballing, logarithmic rise from about thirty-five to ninety years, first described by B. Gompertz in 1825.

There are many theories about the reasons for the dramatic changes in the mortality curve after thirty-five. One group of theories favors the notion that we each have a "bank" of vitality upon which we can draw, but the "savings account" is limited in size. According to this idea, when there has been a sufficient amount of minor damage of various kinds, the store of vitality falls below the level necessary to sustain life.

There is considerable evidence of progressive decline in man's physiological functioning, from age thirty on, which parallels the increased probability of dying. These declines may be seen in such diverse measurements as the conduction velocity of nerve, basal metabolic rate, cardiac output, breathing capacity, and kidney output. Presumably these changes hamper the body's ability to roll with the punches delivered by bacteria, viruses, heat, cold, a charging tiger, or a wildly driven automobile. The threats to man have changed in character with the passage of time—in 1900 dinosaur wounds were no longer a cause of death, but pneumonia, influenza, tuberculosis, and the infectious diarrheas and dysenteries were. Today, the leading causes of death are heart disease, cancer, and stroke, but the Gompertz curve has the same general shape it had in 1825.

There have been attempts to measure the lethal impact of various stresses on laboratory animals of different age. If one takes a mouse or rat and bleeds him, his chance of surviving a given loss of blood diminishes as he gets older. The same is true for his ability to swim until exhausted or to survive a dose of radiation. But this correlation with age is by no means universal. With different drugs, for example, sometimes young rodents are most susceptible to the toxic effects, sometimes the old, and sometimes the middle-aged ones.

The finding of physiological declines in functioning with age has unfortunately implied the gloomy inevitability of "wear and tear."[1] Yet we must remember that arteriosclerosis was once considered irreversible in its onset and its progression with age, while today these changes in blood vessels are more popularly considered the result of such environmental factors as diet and stress. Studies at the Philadelphia Zoological Garden have shown coronary-artery disease in mammals and birds to be less

---

[1] This idea is reinforced by the knowledge that the "death rate" of motor cars is similar to that of wild-type fruit flies.

associated with age than with some of the social changes contingent on attempts to assemble and maintain breeding stocks, with the introduction of new captives, with proximity of males or females of the same species, or with the interaction of the animals with keeper personnel.

Descriptively, there are data on the apparent effect of aging on every organ in the body. The skin acquires telltale wrinkles, roughness, moles, and warts. There is a loss of hair. The teeth tend to deteriorate and to fall out or be extracted, primarily because of peridontal disease. There is a decreased sensitivity to sound, light, tastes, and smells. The digestive juices tend to diminish, and the large intestine develops outpocketings in its wall—so-called diverticulosis. Whereas death is rarely due to a wearing-out of the digestive system, failure of the circulation is a common cause of demise, as the brain, heart, or kidneys are deprived of their blood supply.

The brain is unique among the organs of the body in its correlation with longevity. Sacher has analyzed the maximum life span, brain weight, and body weight of more than a hundred species of mammals and has come up with an equation that satisfactorily represents most of the data:

$$\text{Life Span} \propto \frac{[\text{brain weight}]^{2/3}}{[\text{body weight}]^{2/9}}$$

In other words, life span is directly proportional to brain weight and inversely proportional to body weight. The formula holds for shrews and whales, rodents and primates. For example, man weighs about as much as the white-tailed deer or the mountain lion, but has a brain seven to ten times larger than the brains of the other two species, almost exactly the factor predicted by the equation on the basis of the respective life spans.

What happens to the cells that make up our organs? There is increasing irregularity in the arrangement of cells as an individual grows older, along with a greater variability of nuclear size and an accumulation of pigment in certain cells. There is, as well, a loss of cells. But it is not possible to ascribe the failure of individual organs solely to this. The dramatic decline in the intact aging organism becomes less impressive as the system is broken down into smaller and smaller components. The change in the whole organism greatly exceeds the sum of the changes at the subcellular level.

For more than half a century, it has been popular scientifically to assume that development and aging are, if not identical, at least inextricably linked in a cause-and-effect relationship, and that death is the price we pay for differentiation and organization. Yet no causal relationship has thus far been demonstrated between development and senescence. It is true that a structure must develop before it disintegrates, and that animals of finite body size show a progressive decrease in growth rate as they mature, but this is hardly convincing evidence in support of the hypothesis. In the case of mobile organisms, specific size is probably dictated as much by the physics of running or flying as by the tendency to age. In addition, the cessation of organismal growth does not rule out the regular renewal of subcellular structures for indefinite periods of time. The cells of the human epidermis, intestinal epithelium, and bone marrow might in fact be considered immortal, since they show a continuous regenerative activity during life.

A number of observations suggest the operation of hereditary factors in longevity. The life span of children is positively correlated with that of their parents, and the life spans of identical twins are more closely similar than those of fraternal twins. It has also been possible to change the longevity of mice by selective breeding, and in the fruit fly and other species, hybrids tend to live longer than their purebred parents—the phenomenon of "hybrid vigor," a descriptive term that sounds so impressive that one is sometimes tempted to forget that it explains nothing.

With our increasing preoccupation with the effects of radiation, scientific attention has focused on the parallelism between aging and the biological impact of ionizing radiation. Animals subjected to sublethal doses of radiation die prematurely in what looks like an acceleration of natural aging. Chromosomal aberrations in mice increase as a function both of age and of exposure to radiation, and fragmentary data on survivors of the Hiroshima atomic blasts indicate accelerated aging of their connective tissue.

Diet has also been implicated as a cause of aging. If white rats have their caloric intake restricted enough to retard development, it is possible to double the life span of the dieting animals, and such underfeeding and overfeeding experiments as have been performed on other species tend to support the rat data. In man, also, overweight seems to be correlated with a shortening of life span.

A provocative theory of aging is the autoimmune one. This postulates that the immune mechanisms that usually protect the body against foreign cells go berserk after a while and begin to attack the normal host cells, as abnormal protein induces antibodies with enough cross-reactivity to normal proteins so that damage multiplies beyond the original "hit." The evidence is sketchy so far, although several important life-shortening diseases, such as cancer and diabetes, are thought by some to be autoimmune diseases, and experimentally produced immune disease in young animals is characterized by changes that seem to resemble those of aging.

As an evolutionary process, aging may have positive survival value for the species in several ways. Immortality may be a luxury that most species cannot afford. If senescent individuals compete successfully with their offspring for food, space, and energy, the reproductive capacity of the younger individuals (and thus of the species) may be threatened.

But maturity—short of immortality—can benefit a species. This is most clearly evident in man because of the evident contributions of older individuals to the society, but a quick death is not necessarily the rule even for postreproductive males and females of subhuman[2] species. The Norway rat and the grasshopper *Schistocerca*, for example, spend on the average from one third to one half the life span in postreproductive sterility. It is not clear how a population of rats or insects benefits from the presence of superannuated individuals, but there is no *a priori* reason to consider man unique in profiting from the presence of living ancestors.

Sociologists and psychologists have been interested in what happens psychologically to the aging person in the face of waning physiological powers. Some individuals obviously try to preserve the illusion of unflagging capabilities—the aging movie star, for example, whose trousers get tighter, sports jackets jauntier, cars smaller and faster, with each new wife younger than the last.

Others, more realistic, regroup their physical and mental forces, either doing the same things at an easier pace or giving up some activities so as to carry on others at full throttle. For too many, especially at forced retirement, there is a retreat into pointless leisure, a pursuit of trivial, frivolous, unsatisfying activities that are a grotesque parody of "fun" but are chosen in preference to the life of reading, contemplation, and philosophical speculation which is atypical in our society.

The aged person is not helped in his adjustments by the many threats to his self-esteem. In Western cultures, the elderly are not generally the dominant generation and are likely to be treated with hostility or at best a lack of consideration. Our society tends to worship youth, slimness, vigor. The aged worker is forced from his job at some arbitrary time, unrelated to his powers or contributions, thus losing at once an important source of income, satisfaction, "busy work," and esteem. Spouse and friends die off, leaving a void and the pain of loneliness. Illness, when it comes, is often more serious and devastating than for the younger man and is particularly heartbreaking when the disability brings with it the realization that

2 Do birds refer to us as subavian?

one's children or relatives may not wish the bother of taking back into the home a formerly acceptable oldster after the need for hospitalization is over.

In what ways can the physician help the aged to live more comfortable and more meaningful lives? Many look to medical science to extend man's life beyond his present expectations. Dr. Robert R. Kohn of Western Reserve University has estimated that if people could be kept from developing cancer, or if all cancers could be cured, the life expectancy of adults would be increased only by one to three years. If adults could be freed of atherosclerosis, Kohn estimates that man could expect about seven more years of life. Such figures are of course highly speculative, since diseases are not necessarily discrete entities, but may be interrelated processes. An old person saved from atherosclerosis might be more susceptible to death from influenza or pneumonia and be carried off by another servant of death without making any net gain in life span. What may be in view, even in the event of spectacular medical advances, is less a major stretching of the average life span than the enabling of more people to live the "maximum" life span already enjoyed by some of our aged, so that, in the words of the Book of Job: "Thou shalt come to thy grave in a full age, like as a shock of corn cometh in in his season."

How far we are from solving a riddle like atherosclerosis may help provide both perspective and humility about our chances of conquering this major killer. The present confusion as to theories of its causation and proposed solutions may be suggested by a composite picture by Dr. Gordon S. Myers of Boston of the type of individual with a low risk of developing atherosclerosis or coronary-artery disease:

> An effeminate municipal worker or embalmer, completely lacking in physical or mental alertness and without drive, ambition or competitive spirit; who has never attempted to meet a deadline of any kind; a man with poor appetite, subsisting on fruits and vegetables laced with corn and whale

oil; detesting tobacco, spurning ownership of radio, television or motor car; with full head of hair but scrawny and unathletic appearance, yet constantly straining his puny muscles by exercise. Low in income, blood pressure, blood sugar, uric acid and cholesterol, he has been taking nicotinic acid, pyridoxine, and long-term anticoagulant therapy ever since his prophylactic castration.

Our ignorance is also reflected in the uncertainty about the merits of lowering serum cholesterol concentrations. Many believe that doing this by any means—diet, hormones, or chemicals—will prevent heart attacks, but there is no convincing evidence that this is so. The hypothesis seems reasonable enough, but many reasonable-sounding things have proved to be nonsense when put to the test. The National Institutes of Health are spending millions of dollars to tackle the question in huge field trials. The trials will be complicated—more than fifty hospitals and 8,000 volunteers who have had one heart attack will eventually be involved in the national drug trial—and tedious (they will last at least five years), but without such an experiment we will never know whether the lowering of serum cholesterol after a heart attack has the slightest merit.

Despite our ignorance, there is a great deal the doctor can do for the aged. The profession, however, must alter its thinking in regard to prolonged illness. The permanently disabled and the chronically ill are in general objects of prejudice and discrimination in our society. Physicians share these prejudices, manifesting them in a reluctance to participate in the care of such patients.

Dr. Ewald W. Busse, director of the Center for the Study of Aging at Duke University, has said:

> There are few physicians who are capable of dealing with large numbers of chronically ill persons with sustained enthusiasm. . . . The physician's evaluation of himself as an individual capable of reducing or eliminating pain and restoring function

is apt to suffer when he cannot see clearly the patient's improvement as the result of his efforts.

The physician's self-esteem is also very much influenced by how much he is liked and appreciated by his patients. The chronically ill person who is frustrated by his slow progress is not likely to express gratitude to the physician for his help. In fact, the patient frequently indicates to the physician that he is dissatisfied with his treatment.

The older patient, with his multiple and recurring problems, has a great need—at present rarely met—for continuing, integrated medical care. His hospital experiences are not usually isolated, self-limited illnesses, and the urgency of his health needs will vary tremendously. There must therefore be a smoothly geared mechanism for rapidly admitting the chronically ill person to hospitals for "acute" medical care as well as for quickly facilitating transfer to the home, or a rehabilitative facility, or a long-term custodial facility as the needs change. This requires a much closer liaison between general hospitals, "chronic" hospitals, halfway homes, nursing homes, and home-care programs than now exists.

Acute general hospitals are often poorly equipped to handle chronic disease problems of this sort. A stroke patient admitted there may rapidly develop fearsome bedsores or limb contractures because the doctors and nurses have little experience with the needs of such patients. Chronic hospitals, on the other hand, are all too often third-rate custodial facilities with staffs that are badly deficient in numbers, quality, or both; patients become pathetic vegetables waiting to die, as remote from imaginative attention as they are from the outside world.

Many of our nursing homes have low standards of care. There has been a lot of jockeying for position by different organizations in attempts to remedy the situation, but little real progress in the establishment of adequate criteria for accreditation. Since there are more than 13,000 nursing homes listed by the American Nursing Home Association and many more unlisted, and since it has been estimated that more than 1,000,000 citizens have need of their services, the health of vast numbers of chronically ill is at stake.

In 1962, tentative standards for nursing-home accreditation were approved by a joint commission sponsored by the American Hospital Association, the American Medical Association, the American College of Surgeons, and the American College of Physicians. The AMA subsequently vetoed the plans, however, and joined the American Nursing Home Association to set up a separate accreditation service. Recriminations filled the air. The AMA was accused of selfish motives, the AHA of dictatorial rigidity. The splintering meant fragmentation, increased cost, and decreased quality of patient care, because of the elimination of the AHA from meaningful interaction with the doctors and the nursing homes. How Medicare will affect the nursing homes is not as yet clear, although some experts lugubriously predict that as many as half our nursing homes may fail to meet reasonable standards.

Whatever the standards, and whichever the appropriate accrediting agency, the standards will still need to be implemented. This will require men—doctors with the talent, experience, imagination, dedication, and energy to coordinate the acute, chronic, rehabilitative, and home medical services appropriate to the patient's wants. The community must find and hire these physician-administrators, and the latter must be able to achieve working relationships between agencies, groups, and individuals that may appear superficially incompatible. They must be of a caliber, in background and performance, to command the respect of both the profession and the lay community.

It is not only hospitals and nursing homes that are poorly designed to care adequately for the aged. Our homes are a serious threat to the older person. Most fatal accidents in the home involve people over sixty-five years of age. Burns and falls are responsible for many of these, and much of the trouble could be prevented. Our staircases are too steep, without adequate handrails, and badly lit. Chairs are often not high enough and lack easily grasped arms. Floors are too polished. Beds are not the right height. Bathrooms are slippery, lack steps and built-in handles for getting in and out of the bath. Toilets are low and lack nearby handles to provide support. Kitchen shelves and cupboards are either too high or too low. Devices are needed to prevent pans from being knocked off the stove and for taking hot dishes out of the oven and transporting them to the table. Most of these hazards are neither mysterious nor difficult to prevent; what is needed is a public awareness of the problems and a desire to solve them.

In his functioning as a practitioner, the doctor has to remember constantly that rules that hold for young adults may be completely inappropriate for the geriatric population. In medical diagnosis, for example, doctors are usually well advised, in the younger age groups, to use Occam's razor—the principle that one should not invoke any more assumptions or entities than the minimum necessary to explain a situation. This philosophical rule of thumb, dating back to the fourteenth century, has been viewed over the years as reflecting such diverse forces as God's will, esthetic principles, and laziness, but its appeal to the physician is simply based: it seems to work well in most acute medical problems. In the aged, however, or even in the young with chronic disease, Occam's razor may serve only to cut the patient's lifeline. Such patients rarely suffer from only one condition, and to insist on one diagnosis to explain all the symptoms usually means missing an important facet of the problem.

Dr. David Seegal, Professor of Medicine at Columbia University's College of Physicians and Surgeons, has written on "The Trap of the Pigeonholed Diagnosis":

> . . . the trust given to him by the long-term patient demands a vigilance beyond that of managing the original illness. Although his diagnosis on the first few visits was correct and

the therapeutic regimen exemplary, over the years the busy doctor may be lulled into a comfortable acceptance of the status quo of the diseases in his charge. The disciplined physician of record, however, will avoid many of the traps of the pigeonholed diagnosis by adopting realistic methods for the detection of the subtle beginnings of new disease in the chronically ill under his care. Performance of this duty may benefit the patient and prevent the bitter experiences which each of us has known in the past while hibernating with the original diagnosis.

The aged patient may be caught in other semantic traps. One is the awful word "senility," which covers everything from a dementia secondary to vascular lesions of the brain or neuronal atrophy, to frailty and drug intoxication. It is often used as a substitute for thorough diagnostic and therapeutic measures. The elderly, for example, not infrequently suffer from melancholia. Their depressions may be of various kinds and the remedial measures must be appropriate to the cause. Some patients need only companionship, or hope, or friendship. Others need nourishment, treatment of somatic conditions, or antidepressant drugs. Still others need to have sleeping pills or other medications stopped. None of these measures is provided by a doctor's hopeless, helpless acceptance of melancholy in the aged as the expected result of senility.

Elderly patients are more likely than younger patients to develop complications in the hospital, and the doctor must be on the alert to prevent or treat them. Studies have shown that as many as three fourths of geriatric patients develop such complications, especially respiratory infections, which are often fatal. Pneumonia in the elderly is often undramatic in onset —perhaps only a poor appetite, or pallor, or a slight rise in respiratory rate, or a little fever. Other problems include urinary-tract infections, drug reactions, and injuries sustained from falls.

In the doctor's efforts at health care he must not gamble

with the vitality of the elderly patient by quickly subjecting him to more tests and treatments than he can tolerate with reasonable safety. Doctors are apt to forget how debilitating a rapid-fire X-ray workup can be, for example. A patient is admitted to a hospital with a vague story of belly pain. The physician, rightly concerned with making a diagnosis as soon as possible and keeping hospital costs down for his patient, orders a long list of X rays: a gallbladder series, X rays of the esophagus, stomach, upper intestine, and kidneys, a barium enema, possibly even a series of films of the lower small intestine. Most of these procedures have deleterious effects on the elderly. Some require restriction of food, drink, or both for as long as thirty-six hours before the procedure. Some require castor oil and cleansing enemas before the X rays, and similar measures may be required to clean the barium out of the intestine after the films are taken. On the day of each X-ray examination, there is usually little or no intake of food or liquid while the patient waits—often for many hours—for the films to be taken, and then for additional hours until the pictures are completed. It is not unusual—even if all the films are satisfactory and no repeats are needed—for a patient to go the better part of a week in a state of relative dehydration and starvation. Even a healthy young patient suffers discomfort; the sick oldster whose circulation, heart, kidneys, or brain are barely compensated in the best of circumstances may be pushed over the brink into insufficiency of one sort or another.

On the other hand, it is not necessary for the physician to deny the elderly patient the benefit of needed therapy for serious conditions. The operating-room schedules of all major hospitals are filled with aged patients in their sixties and seventies, and even octogenarians and nonagenarians can successfully undergo major surgery. There are no absolute age limits to surgery, although the physiological age of the patient seems important in predicting risk. What the aged do need, however, is meticulous preoperative preparation, experienced and judicious surgery and anesthesia, and diligent postoperative care. With a smoothly working team of medical and paramedical personnel aware of the special problems of the aged, surgery need not be a fearful or dangerous experience.

One of the lessons the doctor must learn is to be humble in the goals he sets for his geriatric patient. Dr. Alfred Worcester described the problem with feeling:

> In the first year of my practice I undertook the care of a rich old man; misshapen by *arthritis deformans*. I made notes of his history; I examined his body and his excretions; and then I ordered for him the treatment that in those years was according to Hoyle. As his pulse was irregular I cut off his tobacco. I did not allow him even the meats that he depended upon; and in place of his gin I gave him nauseous draughts of salicylates. When a few days afterwards he complained that he must have relief, I cruelly answered that I should make my visits only as often as I thought necessary, and that either the treatment I had ordered was to be continued or another physician could be summoned. The old man managed to live through the winter. Before he died he gave me this lesson. He had called for my help, he said, because of his suffering, not because he expected or even wanted to be cured. In spite of his confession of life-long dependence upon alcohol, I had taken that away and also the comfort of even his pipe. I had changed his diet from what he liked to what he loathed, and worst of all, when he wanted the encouragement of frequent visits, I had refused him even that boon. He was too proud, he said, not to obey his physician's orders, but he wanted me to know how much more miserable I had made the last year of his life. My only atonement has been in never again making just such an egregious blunder; and I report it in the hope that my younger brothers will never make the mistake of treating their aged patients as if their rejuvenation were possible.

Doctors might well take the lead in trying to re-educate society as to the role the aged can play in the world's affairs.

Since the days of Bismarck, it has been traditional for society to act as if sixty-five years of age marks a dreadful moment when capacities suddenly deteriorate and a formerly useful citizen becomes a candidate for the junk heap. Some union wage pacts indeed aim for still-earlier retirement—voluntary to be sure—but designed to get older workers out of the plants.

While there is no intention to suggest that people must be made to work forever, it would seem highly desirable, both for the aged and for society, to be flexible in the matter of age and performance. All the scientific data available testify to the continuity of the aging process. The age of sixty-five may have a meaning for retirement schemes; it has no medical basis as a cutoff point. It takes imagination, however, to create workable techniques for flexible retirement. Dr. Reubin Andres has suggested that it may be less traumatic to retire at a time when colleagues express admiration at the preservation of faculties than to be forced to retire because of deterioration.

Even the most superficial view of fields where men are not considered aged at any particular time reveals the remarkable productivity and wisdom of some men in their seventies and eighties. In art there are such names as Michelangelo, Monet, Renoir, Degas, Rodin, Matisse, Rouault, Vlaminck, Chagall, Braque, and Picasso. Titian may have been one hundred when he died. In music it is characteristic for teachers, performers, and conductors to be active long beyond the age of sixty-five, the phenomenon manifesting itself in recent years in such persons as Toscanini, Stokowski, Stravinsky, Monteux, Beecham, and Casals. Politics, the church, and the law show a similar disdain for age limits—consider Adenauer, Churchill, De Gaulle, Pope John XXIII, and an army of U.S. Senators, Congressmen, and Supreme Court Justices.

C. P. Snow has said:

> What people need is not just to be kept alive. What people need primarily is self-respect, the certainty that they belong

to the community of human beings. This is a feeling which goes on right to the end of one's life. I've never seen any aging person for whom it wasn't real, acute, and imperative. Can we really afford to throw away the abilities of our people simply because they are 60, 65, or 70 years old?

It is my belief that society will, in large part, get from the aged what it expects from them. The history of education provides abundant evidence that the young are usually up to achieving a great deal more than we give them credit for. A comparison of the public-school curriculum today and that of fifty years ago is a sobering lesson. In times of disaster or war, the energies of men surpass the performance expected of them in their ordinary daily lives. If we expect people to fall apart at sixty-five, many of them will obligingly do so. On the other hand, if we expect continued productivity, advice, and wisdom from the elderly, it is much more likely that we will get them and that society will benefit.

Our attitudes will help decide whether aging is simply a progressive debilitation or a process that adds new dimensions to life. Meanwhile, we can try to make each moment as fruitful and as meaningful as possible. A distinguished physician once remarked, "Life is sweet, but is it long enough?" A young woman present quickly rejoined with: "Life is long, but is it sweet enough?"

13

Preparing for Death

I T IS extraordinarily difficult to define some of the most important phenomena pertaining to the human condition.
We all believe we know what we mean by "love," "pain," or
"sleep"—but how are these states to be explained to a being
from another world who has never slept or felt pain, or who
wishes to know what emotions fill the heart of a young lover or
a mother holding her newborn child? Death, at first consideration a remarkably straightforward event, is another phenomenon that eludes precise limits. In 1966 Dr. Esther Ammundsen,
director of the Danish National Health Service, urged assembled experts from forty nations to draft a model law that would
provide a definition of death that would be legally and morally
acceptable.

In primitive cultures, death was decided by holding a
feather or polished stone before the mouth of the individual to
confirm the disappearance of the spirit—that is, the lack of
breath. Medicine men, in anticipation of modern mouth-to-
mouth resuscitation techniques, often tried to blow the spirit
back into the body, with occasional success. Today, a patient
is called dead when the heart and lungs no longer function,
but this definition is obscured by our newfound ability to sup-

port the circulation and respiration by artificial means. We can use machines to breathe for a person who lacks spontaneous respiratory activity, and we can pump the blood for those whose hearts have stopped.

The World Health Organization defines death as the permanent disappearance of life, without the chance of resuscitation. But at what precise moment does this occur? Because of the considerations already mentioned concerning heart and lung function, and because we ordinarily equate meaningful life with a functioning central nervous system, attention has shifted to the brain as the indicator of life. When brain function ceases, the electroencephalogram shows flat-line recordings instead of the usual active electrical squiggles popularly known as brain waves. The French Academy of Medicine has officially pronounced that death occurs with either the irrevocable loss of function of an indispensable organ or a progressive degeneration leading to the physiologic death of such an organ. Death of the brain was accepted as the most prominent function. But no one, however expert he may be in reading electroencephalograms, is able to say exactly when the brain is destroyed—how long the EEG tracing must be a straight line before a person can be declared dead.

Traditionally, scientific dogma has maintained that the brain can survive only three to five minutes without blood flow, but recently a young California woman who had sustained a ruptured heart in an auto accident recovered rapidly and completely following emergency surgery, despite the fact that twenty-one minutes of complete circulatory arrest had elapsed. Clearly, it is impossible to be exact in these matters, and one can only speculate as to what will be considered death in the year 2000, when for all we know that bizarre trick so beloved of science-fiction writers—exchanging one brain for another—may be technically possible.

One legal area in which it is important for the doctor to be able to pinpoint the moment of death is in cases where murder or manslaughter is suspected, when the timing of the fatal injury may be important to the detection of the crime or the rejection of an alibi. This is a problem within the province of the forensic medical specialist, who utilizes autopsy evidence to help fix the time of death, but in other cases it may be necessary to decide when an individual actually under observation is passing from the land of the living into the land of the dead. For example, in some jurisdictions, if someone dies of an injury later than a year and a day after the injury was inflicted, the law presumes that his death resulted from some other cause, and no indictment for murder or manslaughter is possible. The increasing ability of medicine to practice "spare-parts" surgery will put a premium on the rapid removal of organs from a body after death, but the doctor is subject to serious legal risk if the presence of death is not clear, since to hasten the death of anyone, even a person whose death is imminent, is still a homicide.

There are also potential tax implications in the determination of the time of death. Estate tax, for example, may be levied upon gifts made within the three-year period preceding the death of the donor, since under federal law it is presumed that gifts within that period were made "in contemplation of death" and, unless the presumption is rebutted, the gifts are included in the estate for tax purposes. Wealthy individuals may make substantial gifts to their relatives to avoid estate tax, and conceivably a day or week off in deciding when death occurs may determine whether the gift comes within the three-year period. The ghoulish possibility exists that a dying man (or his relatives) may ask that he be kept alive artificially for a prolonged time for the sole purpose of avoiding taxes.[1]

The time or order of deaths also may have important substantive effects upon the devolution of property. It may be quite important to know when close relatives, such as husband and wife, die. If both husband and wife are fatally injured in the same accident and the husband dies first, the wife would

[1] Professor Keith Simpson of Guy's Hospital recently told me of just such a case.

usually inherit his property for the short time before her own death, and such property would ultimately pass to her relatives or to persons entitled under her will. If the wife dies first, her property will usually descend, through the counterpart process, to the husband's side of the family. The order in which the parents die may determine whether the bulk of the estate is subjected to death taxes once or twice (usually with some credit for property previously taxed). If the exact circumstances are not known, in some jurisdictions the law presumes that the younger person survived the elder.

Although the doctor has great difficulty in trying to predict how much life remains for people seriously ill with an apparently fatal illness, many physicians find it difficult not to be oracular; they gravely hold forth at the patient's bedside for the benefit of the relatives, medical students, nurses, or anyone willing to listen. Such prognostic ability would be most helpful in many situations, since both the sick patient and his relatives may have to make important plans, but the art of prognosis is an elusive one, and many an embarrassed doctor has failed to outlive the patient whose immediate doom he prophesied.

During my medical-school days, I was much impressed by a story about one of our most distinguished professors. As a young but not inexperienced physician working in the clinic of a major hospital, he had occasion to see a twenty-year-old woman who was found to have essentially nonfunctioning kidneys. The compassionate business house at which she worked asked how long the patient might be expected to live, were she allowed to continue employment with very light duties. After a comprehensive evaluation, the doctor, along with the other kidney experts in the clinic, expressed the fear that it would not be long. A year later the same form letter was received again and answered in the same way. After four more years of this correspondence between hospital physicians and the employer, the patient finally died.

Even so dreaded a disease as cancer has the most variable

of courses. With breast cancer for which no treatment of any kind is given, the average survival of patients with different degrees of histologic change ranges from twenty-two to forty-seven months. But these mean figures hide the fact that within a given histologic group, as determined by the degree of wildness of the cells on microscopic examination, the survival may range from less than half a year to four, ten, or fifteen years. Although lung cancer ordinarily carries a dismal prognosis, 5 per cent of those afflicted live five years or longer after diagnosis. The literature contains reports of more than 1,000 cases of spontaneous regression of cancer of all sorts. Even where questionable cases are ruled out because of inadequate information, there are still a sizable number of patients considered by cancer experts to show spontaneous disappearance of what appears to be typical malignant disease. These unexpected occurrences point up the need for caution before writing off even the most severely ill patient, just as they reveal the danger in ascribing beneficial results to unorthodox therapeutic measures because of isolated "cures."

In years past, preparation for death was an accepted and sober act, usually taking place at home and more directly concerned with religious faith and one's family than with hospitals or physicians. Today the physician has become for many the one authoritative figure inevitably concerned with death and dying. Unfortunately, medical education does not provide adequate training to deal with the various complicated problems connected with death. Physician surveys reveal that few doctors believe that their approach to the patient with terminal disease owes anything to medical training. Furthermore, doctors disagree markedly concerning what such patients should be told. There is also considerable difference between the way physicians would like to be treated if they were themselves dying and the way they treat their patients.

The majority of doctors usually do not inform patients that they are facing a terminal illness, despite pious pronouncements to the effect that one cannot lie to patients about such matters and that most patients either know they are dying or welcome the opportunity to discuss the problem. In a Chicago survey, however, most doctors wished to be told if *they* were ill, because "I am one of those who can take it" or "I have responsibilities." (Interestingly, most of the doctors said that they were neither more nor less likely to tell physician patients than other patients.) These doctors also indicated that their policies would not be swayed by research on these questions, and some felt that no research into this area should even be done. Various studies indicate that while 70 to 90 per cent of doctors favor not telling the patient, 77 to 89 per cent of patients would wish to be told if they were dying.

While it is often assumed that the fear of death is almost universal, one wonders whether or not such fear actually results from our society's attitude toward death. Since we are impressed from youth onward that life is a beginning and death an end, it is not surprising that many view death as a horror and a void. Paradoxically, the prospect of death is less grim not only for those who believe firmly in an afterlife but for atheists —it is those with a lukewarm, wishy-washy attitude toward religion who have the most difficult time.

Some individuals, who assess life in terms of accomplishments and fulfillment, may fear death because they have not been successful in their own eyes or in the eyes of their survivors or of God. Almost everyone will want a dignified death in which the significance of the individual is not lost, much as Willy Loman's wife in *Death of a Salesman* insisted that Willy was dying psychologically, bit by bit, and that "attention must be paid."

While systematic studies of the dying have been limited, it is evident that in both children and adults with fatal disease, problems of apprehension, depression, and symptomatology need more attention than they have received. Dying patients are usually willing to discuss freely their awareness of dying, often without great emotional disturbance. Those who are suffering physically are more likely to be disturbed than those who are not—one reason why it is important to pay attention to the control of somatic symptoms. During the weeks to months or years before death, there may be a good deal of pain or anxiety or other complaints amenable to therapy, including the use of drugs. The act of dying is itself rarely distressful, because many people lose consciousness for the last hours or days before death.

In guiding the patient through his terminal illness, a number of important considerations must be kept in mind. The doctor must see to it that everything that might reasonably be done to effect a cure and to make the patient comfortable has been done. If other medical talents might be helpful they should be consulted, if only to reassure the patient during his lifetime and the family after death that all that could have been done was in fact done. At the same time, needless visits to a long list of other doctors or clinics should be discouraged, since the only result is likely to be a series of bills that will impoverish the survivors.

The dying patient must be treated no less individualistically than the living. A patient with no close relatives who is at the end of his financial resources and is spiritually prepared to die may be more concerned with the quality of the days remaining than with their number. Another patient, with grievous financial responsibilities, may prefer to keep working as long as possible, regardless of the physical suffering involved. A third person may wish only to be kept free of pain, desiring a death that is dignified and not prolonged.

The doctor must honestly communicate to the patient that his estimates are based on probabilities, not certainties. How detailed the explanation must be depends on the patient's personality. Some patients wish only the simplest of statements, others as full a story as possible. Many patients, having been told the news, prefer to let the matter drop. Others will prefer to discuss the problem at every opportunity. With all his patients, the doctor must avoid both false optimism and a gloomy pity.

The moment of death is traumatic for all concerned, including the doctor. The family is distraught, emotionally drained and often physically exhausted. The doctor is tired, depressed, and frustrated by his failure. Instead of the omnipotent, omniscient authority figure, he is suddenly just another human, powerless in the face of death. His biological training, his storehouse of scientific facts are of little help at such a moment, whereas it counts a great deal how large and warm a soul he has, how much compassion he can share with those who need it.

The doctor will often receive help from the least expected quarter—the dying man. Many individuals manage to meet the end of life in a manner that does great credit to the human species. The famous surgeon William Hunter, in his last words, said: "If I had strength enough to hold the pen I would write how easy and pleasant a thing it is to die." And Cicero relates, in his *De Senectute*: "Just as apples, when unripe, are torn from trees, but, when ripe and mellow, drop down, so it is violence that takes life from young men, ripeness from old. This ripeness is so delightful to me, that as I approach nearer to death, I seem, as it were, to be sighting land, and to be coming to port at last after a long voyage."

One of the most difficult problems facing the doctor is the prolonged existence of individuals suffering from terminal illness. All doctors sooner or later are charged with the care of a patient in coma, incapable of spontaneous respiration, kept "alive" by a mechanical respirator, with fluids and nutrition being pumped in day and night, but with the patient really dead physiologically and legally dead the moment the respirator is turned off. Such patients do not regain the ability to breathe spontaneously, and an autopsy almost always shows advanced degeneration of the brain. Is there any point in maintaining life in such an individual? If not, is there a difference between not starting the respirator at the very beginning and stopping it once it has started?

Historically, the shortening of a person's life under any circumstances has usually been considered undesirable and illegal. Ecclesiastical opinions as far back as the sixteenth and seventeenth centuries have, however, made a distinction between "ordinary" and "extraordinary" means of preserving life. These authorities have stated that individuals are required to utilize ordinary means of avoiding death, but not extraordinary ones. The difficulty arises in the definition of these words. During the centuries in question, the amputation of a leg or the incision of an abdomen was considered extraordinary. With the coming of modern anesthesia and surgery, however, such procedures became ordinary. Hence what was moral in the seventeenth century became immoral in the nineteenth and twentieth centuries.

Some Catholic authorities have expressed the feeling that persons are bound to use only "natural" aids. Such a position seems difficult to defend, since it would lead to a position wherein modern antibiotics, since they are artificially produced and administered, might be considered unnatural and extraordinary means for preserving life. Modern authorities, while agreeing that something like intravenous feeding is ordinary and not unnatural, nevertheless do not feel that treatment of this sort is obligatory.

Most of these opinions lead to the conclusion that the prolongation of human life per se is not an absolute good, but a relative one. If the ending of a life is preferable to continuation, one must ask in what sense it is preferable. Can we make such decisions without coming to grips with the problem of the meaning of human life itself, and why ultimately human life must be preserved?

The Reverend Joseph Fletcher has suggested the new term "anti-dysthanasia." He uses this word for what he calls indirect euthanasia. By direct euthanasia he would consider acts specifically to end life, such as introducing air into a patient's blood to cause a fatal embolism or administering a fatal overdose of morphine. Indirect euthanasia is "mercifully hastening death or at least mercifully refusing to prolong it." Death is considered thereby to be permitted but not induced. Thus, withholding treatment or stopping it would be allowable, whereas administering an overdose of drug would not.

Legally, there is no way for the physician to hasten death, even if the patient requests it and the family approves of it. Yet the physician is duty-bound and morally justified to relieve suffering. Two recent Swedish cases illustrate the confusion. Both were patients of the same physician. In the first instance, an eighty-year-old woman died when the physician stopped intravenous therapy that had been keeping her alive for five weeks following a massive cerebral hemorrhage. The relatives had consented to stop the treatment. In the second case, a sixty-five-year-old woman in coma, the doctor had told the relatives that the condition was hopeless and asked for the right to end treatment. Both cases came to public attention when the son of the second patient accused the doctor of planning to kill his mother. Sweden's Central Medical Board found the physician guilty in both cases, but in court the judge ruled, in a decision that has been considered a big step toward legalizing euthanasia, that the physician had acted properly both times, and that relatives had the moral right to make decisions as to prolongation of life in such hopeless cases.

Most people who are opposed to euthanasia are unwilling to allow the patient to have a say in the matter. Many patients are incapable of giving permission, because they are in coma or otherwise unresponsive, but what of the patient who has indicated his desire? Ingemar Hedenius, a Swedish philosophy professor, has proposed that healthy people be given the right to sign up for *dödshjälp* ("death help") on their health insurance cards. He divides this death help into passive and active categories. Passive death help is like Fletcher's anti-dysthanasia. Active death help is the administration of pain-killing drugs in such amounts as to shorten life. Hedenius has indicated that he would rather die than suffer immeasurable pain or become a helpless wreck without any prospect of a decent human existence, that he would rather die than usurp a hospital bed with his own meaningless suffering when others might be nursed back to health in that bed, and that he would rather die than have relatives wish him dead in vain and remember him as a distasteful wreck.

The journalist Helen Hill Miller has discussed the same issue as follows:

> As younger persons become accustomed to the sight of terminal illness of the very old, what if they, while still in good health and sound mind, wish to instruct family, physician and the institution where they may one day be after an incapacitating stroke or when deterioration has reached a non-reversible state, that they are not to be maintained in an existence that has lost all significance. Should a properly attested instrument not be accorded the same validity as an individual's last will, likewise prepared in advance with a view to a future contingency?

It seems reasonable for physicians to discuss these contingencies and to consider the possibility of committees made up of appropriate medical and nonmedical members (including perhaps representatives of the patient's family) to decide about euthanasia in certain instances. I do not mean to minimize the difficulties involved. The taking of life is an awesome business. But safeguards are conceivable that could eliminate the danger of the rapacious or guilt-laden relative or the amoral physician. One would have to maintain the individual's dignity as well as the dignity and peace of mind of his family and his physician, but the task need not be an impossible one.

Physicians who oppose euthanasia cite a number of reasons for their stand. One is the possibility that a new cure may be discovered at any moment, a notion impossible to rule out. But there are more cogent reasons, such as the knowledge that the physician is fallible, and that his diagnosis and prognosis may be incorrect. Also, no one is eager to judge whether the quality of a given life is worth maintaining.

Yet, whether he likes it or not, the physician cannot avoid this judgment. He is in essence making a decision about euthanasia whenever he has to order a life-sustaining medication for a terminally ill patient. When different treatments of potentially fatal illnesses are available, such as surgery or radiotherapy or drugs for malignant cancer, the physician will have to decide whether one form of treatment is to be preferred to another. He may have to judge whether a treatment that provides less physical and mental stress but a shorter life may not be better than one that prolongs life to a greater degree but at the cost of great suffering. There is no place for the physician to hide.

Surveys of American physicians show that approximately a third of all doctors feel that euthanasia is justified in the case of a patient in great pain without hope of relief or recovery. (This figure is close to 40 per cent for Protestants and Jews, but only 7 per cent for Roman Catholics.) Similar figures apply to the case of infants born with serious abnormalities and with no chance of a normal life. Indeed, many physicians covertly practice at least indirect euthanasia by making little or no effort to resuscitate a child born with the grossest of congenital anomalies.

The ambivalence of society itself is manifest in certain public treatments of the problem. In the early 1950's, a New Hampshire physician injected air into one of his dying patients, but his only punishment was temporary suspension of license. In 1963 a physician was tried for murder in Liège for complicity with a mother in destroying a thalidomide baby, but was acquitted. A bill was actually once introduced in the New York legislature that would have permitted a patient to apply for euthanasia—the doctor would issue a certification and a committee would be empaneled to consider the petition of the patient.

The ability of the medical profession to decide how and when the ill shall die has been enhanced in a dramatic way by two advances in the treatment of irreversible kidney failure— the so-called chronic-dialysis programs and the transplantation of healthy kidneys from donors. In 1965 a scandal erupted at the famous Karolinska Hospital in Stockholm. While the professor of surgery was away on vacation, a team of physicians at his clinic transplanted a kidney from a dying woman to a man whose kidney function had stopped. The woman was unconscious and could not consent to the removal, but the woman's husband gave his unhesitating approval. The woman was placed in a respirator and died two days after the operation, and the forty-five-year-old man to whom the kidney had been transplanted died within two weeks.

The hospital was racked by controversy. Some physicians on the staff bitterly opposed the procedure, while others, including the absent chief of surgery, approved. The operation was aired on a nationwide television debate, with both physicians and philosophers answering yes to the question: "Have we the right to remove vital organs from a dying person if by so doing we can save another person's life?"

Of the thousands of individuals in the United States who die of chronic renal failure each year, only a small percentage can be sustained alive by the most enthusiastic chronic-dialysis programs. These programs are the culmination of research started in 1913. At that time dogs whose kidneys had been removed were successfully kept alive by passing their blood through a network of tubes that allowed the passage of poisons out of the blood. Some thirty years later a Dutch physician, Willem Kolff, introduced the first practical treatment of a patient with an artificial kidney. These ingenious machines are now widely accepted as a mode of treatment for acute reversible kidney failure, but it is only in the last decade that the same principle has been applied to the patient with permanent renal failure.

These procedures are not without difficulty. Patients have usually returned to the hospital once a week or so to have their blood cleared of its poisons, and many things may go wrong for the patient. (Recently there has been some success in dialyzing patients at home while they sleep, and an ingenious Japanese doctor has dialyzed patients by installing cellophane coils in the home washing machine, a technique now on trial in the United States and elsewhere. Dialysis machines, while expensive, may now also be bought for home use.) With prolonged treatment, the dialysee may suffer infections, neurological disease, disease of the bones, arthritis, hepatitis, gastrointestinal hemorrhage, and pulmonary complications. Many patients, disillusioned with the low level of life available to them with this treatment, become despondent, and some have committed suicide. But others seem to function well and are restored to a productive life.

The cost of these centers is considerable. The Veterans Administration Hospital at Denver estimated in 1965 that per diem costs for treating such a patient come to $70.15, because of the multiple chemical and microbiological procedures required, as well as the needs of the blood bank and the pathology laboratory. The government has allocated millions of dollars to support research on their problem and has set up units at a number of hospitals. In every society, however, money is limited, and a decision has to be made about priorities in funding. In fact, millions for dialysis units means millions kept out of some other health effort.

The establishment of dialysis centers has created logistic and ethical problems for physicians. One is the very decision as to whether a hospital should undertake to provide such a service. Money is not the only consideration. Space and facilities are required, and personnel as well. Many busy and talented researchers have been unwilling to devote a considerable portion of their energies to the supervision of such units, feeling that society is in the long run better off if their efforts are put toward discovering ways of preventing irreversible renal disease.

Serious problems exist even after one has decided to undertake such a program. How should one pick the patients, since at present there are more candidates than can be handled? Some groups leave the matter to chance on a first come, first served basis,[2] others use lay committees representing the community to judge whose life should be saved. On what considerations should the selection be based—the potential value of the subject to society, the burden he leaves behind when he dies, or what? What happens if the patient after a time no longer fulfills the original criteria?

In general, there is agreement that dialysis should ideally be a preparation for ultimate renal transplantation. This too presents its problems. Human kidneys for transplantation can be obtained from only three sources. (A fourth possibility, transplants from other species, is still so experimental that as yet it does not deserve to be listed.) The first is from people who have a kidney removed for therapeutic reasons. These are usually not suitable because the very reasons that require the kidney to be removed also make it not useful for transplantation. The second source is from living volunteers. The risk of donating a kidney is small but real. Although it is not likely that the loss of a kidney will greatly curtail one's life span, there is always the remote possibility of an operative death. When, therefore, is it appropriate to accept a kidney from a living volunteer? Obviously the donor must be in good health and must have two kidneys, each of which is normal. In addition, however, he must be fully aware of the risks he is accepting and the donation must be voluntary. He must also be aware of the very considerable chance that his sacrifice may turn out to be of little or no benefit to the patient.

It has been suggested that there are no serious barriers to

---

[2] Legally and ethically, a random choice by lot among those medically suitable would probably be most compatible with precedents in other situations.

the donation of kidneys, since if a man may sacrifice his life for his colleagues in peace or war, then why may he not sacrifice a kidney? But there are problems, including legal traditions in many parts of the world that a person may not maim himself. The situation is least difficult when the patient and the donor are identical twins of adult age, where the prospects of success are excellent and the psychological atmosphere is also very favorable. What to do, however, in the case of twins who are under the age of twenty-one? Can a child really consent to a procedure of this sort? Can the parent consent on his behalf?[3]

A parent who wishes to donate a kidney to his child may be a suitable candidate, after frank discussions of the situation and adequate time for reflection, but the doctor must discourage the parent from doing this out of guilt and emotional confusion. The doctor must also see to it that the parent understands that the prognosis is much less favorable than in the case of transplantation from an identical twin. Similar problems arise in the use of siblings, husbands and wives, and close friends.

The third source of kidneys is from cadavers, and can be a most satisfactory source when properly exploited. Satisfactory kidneys are difficult to obtain, however, since many who die have disease of the kidneys and sometimes the organs are irreparably damaged during the last few hours of life. The kidney deteriorates rapidly after death and is unlikely to function well if the period between the death of the patient and the restoration of the circulation of the kidney after transplantation is more than about three hours. (By contrast, a corneal graft can be delayed for six hours or so with little consequence.) The most suitable subjects are those in whom death has resulted from accidental injury or during a surgical operation, but there is often considerable delay in obtaining permission to remove

---

[3] In one ruling, it was decided that such a twin could contribute a kidney because it would be prejudicial to his psychological well-being not to—an interesting legal gymnastic.

organs in these cases, either because the coroner has to be consulted or because the next of kin are not readily available. Even when the family can be found they are often so upset by their sudden and unexpected loss that they do not understand what is being asked of them.

Furthermore, it is in just this type of case that artificial respiration and cardiac massage may be useful. Either the patient recovers, in which case he is no longer available as a donor, or there comes a time when the decision must be made to switch off the machines and abandon a lost cause. The longer the injured patient is connected to machines, the more his kidneys and other vital organs are likely to deteriorate, so that the doctor may be accused of stopping life solely to achieve the transplant. There has already been a case in Great Britain involving a man whose brain had been irreparably damaged. A kidney was removed from him at surgery while his respiration was sustained. After the kidney was transplanted, the respirator was stopped and the patient declared dead. The surgeon was charged with manslaughter, but the case was dismissed.

People who want their organs to be available after death for purposes of transplantation should make this known to their next of kin, their doctors, and their legal advisers. Recently the states of Virginia and North Dakota have passed legislation giving adults (over twenty-one in Virginia and eighteen in North Dakota) the unchallengeable right to bequeath their bodies and organs for transplantation or other medical procedures. It is to be hoped that other states will follow this lead. We also badly need improved methods of resuscitation to keep to a minimum the deterioration of the kidneys at death, and we need to discover methods of preserving tissues and organs in a healthy state before they are removed from the body. It has been suggested that kidneys might also be obtained from those whose death is the result of judicial execution, but it is doubtful if the few kidneys available from such cadavers are worth the support this might offer to those who still approve the barbaric practice of capital punishment.

An important question is whether medicine by its very success in preserving the weak and the defective is imposing an intolerable burden on society and on its medical services. Will one day all the world become a hospital, as has been predicted, with everyone an ambulatory patient?

Today we can keep people alive who would certainly have died fifty years ago. Such people will grow up and have children and may therefore perpetuate the genetic factors that are responsible for their physical shortcomings. From the eugenic point of view, the most important effects are those of so-called recessive determination, those in which the causative genes must be inherited from both parents if the disease is to become manifest. Although individually these diseases are rare, collectively they are numerous: they include phenylketonuria, galactosemia, cystic fibrosis, and congenital hypogammaglobulinemia. These afflictions result from specific molecular metabolic lesions, and if the victims are kept alive and eventually reproduce the genetic factors responsible will acquire a frequency higher than would be reached were the forces of natural selection allowed to rule.

Obviously we must continue to work toward the prevention and cure of these diseases. Neither society nor medicine can prevent the union of all harmful recessive genes, because all sex cells carry a few—possibly five or six—harmful recessive genes. On the other hand, we know that if two carriers of disease happen to marry each other, one quarter of their children on the average will contract the disease and one half of their children will, like themselves, be carriers. Thus, if we can identify the carriers and discourage them from marrying each other or discourage them from having children if they do marry, the overt incidence of these diseases would diminish or disappear. This does not contraindicate marriage to noncarriers, and merely limits slightly the availability of spouses. This type of genetic detective work and genetic counseling is at least partially possible today and might be a great deal more applicable in the future.

In a sense, however, this process will actually help to promote the spread of the offending gene. It will prevent the outward manifestation of the disease, which depends on the conjunction of two such genes in one person, but it will also remove an obstacle to the spread of the gene, namely the death or infertility of the people who carry it. It has been suggested by Peter Medawar that no one should be dismayed by this prospect. The rate of genetic deterioration brought about by such an approach would be extremely slow, and within the hundreds of years available to us before the impact is felt, solutions in the form of direct intervention via genetic repair processes will perhaps be found to cope with most of these difficulties.

These various considerations illustrate that the approaches taken by the medical profession and society to the problem of death are not immutable. The very act of dying has been so altered in recent centuries as to necessitate a re-examination of our system of moral and societal values. Even euthanasia, so long barred from ethical and legal discussions, is now under scrutiny by many thoughtful scientists and laymen. A review of the past shows that a rigid, dogmatic attitude toward death is historically, scientifically, and morally indefensible. It is a pity, to quote Rostand, that "science has made us Gods before we are even worthy of being men."

Part III

THE INTERFACE
BETWEEN MEDICINE
AND THE LAW

14

Samaritans, Semantics, and Secrecy

THERE IS a fundamental discrepancy between the attitudes of most patients toward the patient-doctor relationship and the legal attitude toward this relationship. Patients in general are ill, suffering from pain or anxiety or other stressful symptoms. They seek help and are usually more than willing to rely implicitly on the physician. Many are completely passive and want the physician to be in absolute control of the situation. It is the minority of patients who look upon the physician-patient relationship as one of mutual participation in the search for health. Yet it is this minority attitude that is embodied in the law, which makes the patient the equal of the doctor and their relationship like a negotiated agreement between equals.

What elements enter into the making of a contract between a patient and his doctor? To begin with, the patient offers to enter into the contract when he consults the doctor in his office, calls him to his home, or visits the hospital to seek care. Second, the physician accepts the offer, either by word of mouth or writing or by initiating treatment. Neither the law nor the doctor's professional code forces him to be an unwilling partner. The law does not require a doctor to care for every patient who wishes to engage his services, and while the ethical code assumes that physicians will refuse to render care only for valid professional reasons, the same code recognizes the right of the physician to refuse to supply care.

The terms of the contract must also be established by the parties. A physician faced, for example, with a Jehovah's Witness who is bleeding but refuses to be given blood or blood products because of religious scruples has several choices available. He may refuse to accept the patient with these restrictions, or he may accept the care of the patient with the understanding that the patient explicitly assumes any hazards resulting from the failure to receive blood and blood products. To be valid the contract must deal with lawful objects. Thus no amount of adherence to the other elements of the contract will make an agreement by a physician to perform an illegal abortion valid.

The parties must be competent to enter into agreement. Someone who is not licensed to administer medical care cannot lawfully contract to render it, and a patient who is not competent cannot lawfully enter into a contract. This latter contingency most commonly occurs with individuals under twenty-one years of age or mentally incompetent.[1] In the case of a child brought to a doctor by a young mother who herself is under twenty-one, the same limit of liability would seem applicable.

In legal jargon, the contract must also involve "the transfer of a lawful object from one of the parties to the other." A physician's services or the promise of such services constitute such consideration, and the promise on the part of the patient to pay the physician's fee is a reciprocal consideration. Once a doctor has rendered service, the patient is obligated to pay, just as the physician is obligated to render service once a patient has rendered payment in advance.

---

[1] There are quasicontractual arrangements that can be made with infants and lunatics, with different limits of liability.

Finally, the contract must be in a form required by law. In most states there is a statute (the "statute of frauds") that specifies those contracts that must be in writing to be enforceable. The agreement involving service by doctors is generally excluded from this category, so that an oral or implied agreement between parties for medical services is customary and enforceable.

Once entered into, such contracts are generally terminated voluntarily by the agreement of both parties. The patient may cease to call upon the physician and engage another physician as he wishes, although any service performed by the doctor up until the time he learns that the patient has decided to terminate the contract is compensable. If a physician wishes to terminate the patient-doctor relationship, he must do so under circumstances that allow the patient to make alternative arrangements if an abrupt termination might endanger his life or health.

Some elements of this contractual relationship run counter, in many instances, to the doctor's ethical code, to society's desires, or to both. Physicians, for example, have become increasingly reluctant to stop and render emergency medical treatment to the victims at the scene of accidents. Doctors are said to fear that malpractice suits will be brought against them by an ungrateful victim or his family. As a result of pressures on this point, the legislatures of forty states have passed laws granting some form of immunity to physicians in this situation; the majority of these laws were enacted since 1960. The Massachusetts statute provides that no licensed physician "who in good faith renders emergency care or treatment" at the scene to automobile-accident victims shall be liable in a suit for damages for any "acts or omissions" in giving such aid. The laws of other states are in many instances broader than that of Massachusetts, granting immunity in any emergency situation.

There is question whether a public need for such laws exists. Not a single suit of this type has reached the appellate level of any jurisdiction in the United States. There have apparently been no trial-court cases in this country, although one action involving a Massachusetts physician has been reported in the Virgin Islands. Statistics on insurance claims also do not indicate this to be an area of significant risk. As a result of these facts, Governor Kerner of Illinois and Governor Rockefeller of New York vetoed so-called Good Samaritan laws, that had been sent to them for their signatures.

In addition to the lack of evidence of excessive risk for Good Samaritan doctors, the medical ethical code states categorically that the physician "in an emergency . . . should render service to the best of his ability." Although a physician who bypasses an accident scene is therefore in fact unethical, only 50 per cent of doctors queried in a survey by the American Medical Association said that they would stop to render aid in an emergency. States that have Good Samaritan laws do not show percentages that differ substantially from those that do not. Thus, either doctors are not aware of the legislation, or they continue to fear liability in spite of the statutes, or they simply don't want to be bothered on their way to business or pleasure.

It is not clear what immunity is actually given by these laws. In general they require that the physician act as a volunteer and without fee. Physicians who do not act gratuitously in such emergency situations may not be granted protection. But what is meant, in these statutes, by rendering care "in good faith"? These laws grant immunity only from suits for "ordinary negligence" and not for "gross negligence" or "recklessness." It is obvious that a plaintiff's attorney could add the adjective "gross" to his complaint and successfully force the physician and his insurance carrier to litigate. Some have argued that such legislation could actually encourage lawyers to plead and prove gross negligence. For doctors concerned more about their reputations than their insurance-claims records, such a development would be most distressing.

While the physician is not legally required at present to

provide medical care, the public shows signs of being increasingly reluctant to allow him such total freedom of action. Rejecting night or emergency calls or refusing to take care of unattractive and demanding patients may evoke unfortunate repercussions. Some years ago a child was struck by an automobile on a corner next to a large building in which many physicians were housed. Someone who had seen the accident tried to engage the services of six separate physicians who were in their offices at the time, but all declined to respond, stating that they were busy with a patient or that their medical specialties were not appropriate to care for the patient. Their actions were publicly condemned and greatly injured the reputation of the medical profession in the community.

In Brooklyn, New York, a doctor had his license suspended for thirty days in 1965 for refusing to treat a postman who had been accidentally shot. In France, a doctor was sentenced to jail, along with six bystanders, for not going to the aid of a man who had been stabbed in a public dance hall. The French Medical Association protested to the Premier and the Minister of Justice, since the doctor contended that he had asked that the man be brought to his home in an ambulance. After other doctors in the Lorraine region went on strike by not answering emergency calls after eight in the evening, the physician was released.

Since medical service in the Armed Forces is obligatory, and since a lawyer may be designated by a court to defend an accused person, the law could also make medical service obligatory. At present, the doctor who withholds his services is in much the same position as the expert swimmer who stands on the riverbank and watches a child drown without making any effort to save him. Neither "expert" is as yet responsible to the law, only to his conscience and public opinion.

The compensation aspect of the patient-doctor contractual agreement has given rise to many arguments. A major source of controversy involves the patient's ability to pay. Some courts refuse to recognize that the wealth of the patient is a factor to consider. They argue that a service is a service no matter who receives it, and like ordinary goods or labor should have a standard value for everyone. Most courts seem to consider it proper for the fee to be fixed according to the patient's financial ability. In part, this is based on the now fading philosophy sometimes referred to as the "Robin Hood school," which stresses that physicians perform many gratuitous services and that they take care of patients who could not possibly compensate the doctor for the care he provides. Presumably in a society that recognizes the right of an individual to contract freely where no public interest is involved, a doctor should be able to place any value on his services in advance of their rendition by agreement with the patient.

It is fascinating that doctors who ordinarily thoroughly enjoy the authoritarian relationship between themselves and their patients are perfectly willing to consider the patient an equal when it comes to financial arrangements for providing health care. The official AMA stand is that the patient should be free to contract and free to make choices, and should reimburse the physician based on the private contractual agreement. If the patient is unable to pay, however, then the doctor no longer considers the patient an equal. Most physicians do not look upon medical care as a right, something to be obtained without suffering indignity. Most of them feel that medical care is like food, clothing, and shelter, and is no more automatically to be obtained than the latter. The average citizen, however, is increasingly unwilling to play the role of grateful serf when he is in need of medical help and cannot afford it.

The legalistics of consent as it pertains to medical research has come to the fore in recent years. Before World War II there was so little human experimentation that people thought about it in terms of *Arrowsmith* or the Walter Reed volunteers, or possibly of mad scientists in horror movies. Three factors brought about a dramatic change. The first was the great availability of research funds from governmental and private sources, with a phenomenal increase in the research establishment. The second was the tremendous growth of the American drug industry, with thousands of compounds manufactured for testing in man. The third was the publicity given to Nazi experiments during the war. This latter research was obnoxious on a variety of counts—the use of condemned prisoners, the inhuman aspects of much of the experimentation, and the trivial scientific merit of most of it.

During the Nuremberg Trials a code was elaborated that rigidly defines the conditions under which human beings can be utilized for research purposes. This code, while it has received considerable publicity, did not have much impact on the performance of research in this country. It was not until the passage in 1962 of the Kefauver-Harris Amendments to the Food and Drug Act that the problem of consent rose clearly into the consciousness of the researchers of the United States. (The legal problem had existed in theory for years.) Section 505 of the act provided that investigators should "obtain the consent of [human beings to whom investigational new drugs are given] or their representatives, except where they deem it not feasible or, in their professional judgment, contrary to the best interests of such human beings."

Many investigators took the phrasing to mean that informed consent was not required when a valid experiment devoid of exceptional risk could not be conducted after obtaining fully informed consent from patients. New regulations issued by Commissioner James Goddard of the Food and Drug Administration in August 1966 indicated that this is not the legal situation. "Not feasible" was stated to be "limited to cases where the investigator is not capable of obtaining consent because of inability to communicate with the patient or his representative." An example is given of the case of a patient in coma whose representative cannot be reached and for whom it is imperative that a drug be administered without delay.

Furthermore, "informed consent" is now defined in great detail. It involves not only the legal capacity of a subject to give consent, but an explanation of "all material information" concerning the drug, the inconveniences and hazards "reasonably to be expected," and the existence of alternative forms of therapy.

It must be recognized that clinical research with new drugs falls into different categories. In one type the relative efficacy of a new agent is evaluated by its impact on the clinical condition of the patient. Here the patient stands to benefit from the trial, and the approach is quite different from the giving of a new drug to volunteer students or prisoners simply to find out how well a drug is tolerated and what doses may be safely employed in the sick. In the second situation, the subject has nothing to gain in regard to his health, and the experimental cards must be laid completely on the table. There is a similar distinction between a patient with congenital heart disease who requires cardiac catheterization to help with the diagnosis and the management of his condition, and a healthy person subjected to catheterization during exercise to study the physiological consequences of such activity.

In the Helsinki Declaration promulgated by the World Medical Association, there is an awareness of the difference between "clinical research combined with professional care" and "non-therapeutic clinical resarch." This declaration, which has been endorsed by the AMA, the American Federation for Clinical Research, the American College of Surgeons, the American Academy of Pediatrics, the American College of Physicians, and other medical groups, is much more flexible in its approach than the new FDA regulations, although the latter refer to the Helsinki Declaration.

It says, for example, that "in the treatment of the sick person, the doctor must be free to use a new therapeutic measure, if in his judgment it offers hope of saving life, reestablishing health, or alleviating suffering. If at all possible, consistent with patient psychology, the doctor should obtain the patient's freely given consent after the patient has been given a full explanation."

While it is not evident how much of the impetus for the new regulations has come from Congressional prodding of the FDA, doubtless some of the force for change derived from the widespread publicity given two events: the injection of cancer cells into some aged residents of a Brooklyn Hospital, and a speech (later published) by Dr. Henry K. Beecher, professor of anesthesia at Harvard. In the first situation, despite the absence of harm to the subjects, the fact that consent was not obtained resulted in disciplinary action by the regents of the University of the State of New York against the doctors involved.

In his indictment, Dr. Beecher compiled a list of fortyeight published examples of research in which the obtaining of consent was not mentioned. He assumed that failure to mention consent in the published report was synonymous with failure to obtain consent—a debatable assumption, since it has not been traditional to list such aspects of experimental protocol in scientific papers. The examples included cases where effective treatment was withheld from patients with typhoid fever, as a result of which 23 patients died needlessly; cases of induction of liver toxicity with a drug in juvenile delinquents and mental defectives; and a variety of experiments involving the sticking of gadgets of various kinds into the heart.

Few would quarrel with Dr. Beecher's request for more candor with experimental subjects, but many wonder about the harmful impact of the new FDA regulations, which go beyond the letter of the 1962 law and disregard the legislative history of the act. Senator Jacob K. Javits, one of the leaders in the original discussion of the consent section, could probably be cited as backing the new interpretation, but not the majority of Congressmen who spoke to the point during the hearings on the bill. Senator James Eastland, for example, stated that "the record should show that the Food and Drug Administration is opposed to it. Furthermore, it is not one of the recommendations the President of the United States made." Representative Oren Harris refused to endorse the consent requirement without discretion to omit consent in some cases. Senator Estes Kefauver himself, prime architect of the 1962 amendments, felt that the consent requirement "would be difficult to enforce and about impossible to police."

It is not clear, for example, how much information should be given a patient with metastatic cancer who has had the first-line standard drugs, is rapidly going downhill, and is therefore a candidate for a brand-new agent. Most physicians would not be willing to lay all these cards on the table.[2] How is one to evaluate a new hypnotic agent in chronic insomniacs who swear that they would not sleep a wink without drugs, but who actually often sleep magnificently (and without risk of side effects) on a placebo capsule—provided they do not know that it is a placebo. Will such patients consent to a placebo trial, even if they are told that the failure of the placebo to induce sleep will result in the prompt administration of a second, standard treatment?

Consider women suffering from postpartum pain. It is not unusual for a placebo to be indistinguishable from standard drugs in this situation. A placebo control is therefore mandatory to allow evaluation of a new agent, because the failure to show a difference between aspirin and the new drug may mean that the new drug is as good as aspirin, or may only indicate that one has picked a population of women who cannot tell a good drug from a bad. The new drug might in fact be better than aspirin, worse, or the same—it is impossible to guess which. But can one explain all this without making the trial pointless?

2 Despite the apparent lack of intent on the part of the FDA to include such cases under the new regulations, many investigators have not read the regulations in this way. The National Cancer Institute, for example, warned all investigators working under their auspices that "the large majority of [incurable cancer] patients will be expected to sign such a consent form."

Few responsible investigators are willing to break the law and risk professional catastrophe for the sake of supplying to the drug industry and to the government the data required to allow rational decisions about the marketing of new drugs. We could revert to older times and perform uncontrolled trials with new drugs, but such trials are generally acknowledged to be substantially less reliable than controlled ones, and competent investigators would refuse to conduct them. If data from uncontrolled trials are to serve as a basis for governmental decision, the FDA will end up approving drugs that are on the average inferior to those we now have. If such data are not to be believed and are disregarded by the FDA, then new drug applications based on the data will have to be rejected. It is unlikely that either alternative is really what the public wants and needs.

I believe safeguards for the patient's welfare and rights are available in the form of review by institutional committees of research protocols and of the conduct of experiments. It is increasingly common for protocols to be scrutinized by a board of scientists at an institution—or even by a mixed lay-professional board including religious and legal representatives—to see that no cutting of ethical corners is contemplated, that no reckless research is planned, that care has been taken to minimize unavoidable risk and to avoid all needless risk, and that there is provision to halt a trial for a given patient at the first suggestion that he is suffering either from the new drug or from the withholding of standard drugs.[3]

Written consent is not ordinarily obtained for that most common and fundamental situation involving drugs—the contractual relation between patient and doctor—and one wonders whether written consent is really necessary for the patient's benefit, as distinguished from the doctor's legal protection. A vague all-purpose written consent form adds little

[3] Such peer review may protect the patient better than informed consent, since some people will volunteer for studies that would be vetoed by the reviewing scientists as too hazardous.

to a verbal discussion with the patient that is as detailed as the situation permits or demands, and it certainly does not substitute for thoughtful face-to-face discussion. If one is to have a detailed written consent form, what is to protect the investigator when something occurs that is not spelled out in so many words? (Even in regard to serious surgical operations, the advice of such legal experts as Burke Shartel and Marcus L. Plant in *The Law of Medical Practice* is to "insist on consent in broad general terms.") If we make clinical investigation less and less like ordinary medical practice and more and more atypical in the type of patient studied, data thus collected may be less and less applicable to the general use of a drug. Surely the less artificial a clinical trial the better, with departures from ordinary clinical practice being only those required from the standpoint of experimental rigor so as to allow one to interpret the data.

Consent implies informed consent. The mere statement to a patient that he is to receive some sort of new compound, without additional information, constitutes an ethical charade. But to obtain informed consent involves many assumptions. It assumes that the investigator knows the risks of giving a drug or performing a given operation, withholding the drug or operation, and the alternative risks from the use of other, older agents or operations that might be used instead. It assumes that the investigator is capable of the exposition required to present this information to the patient, and that the patient is capable of grasping the information. In some areas, such as the use of radioactive diagnostic or therapeutic materials, there is great disagreement even among scientists as to just what the risks of genetic damage or ultimate somatic harm are, and just what a patient can be told.

There is also the possibility that the volunteers' knowledge that they are participating in an experiment will affect the data. As Professor Philip K. Bondy of Yale pointed out:

... a procedure which carries a low risk, if described to a layman who has never seen or heard of such things, is likely to appear a procedure of high risk. For example, cardiac catheterization carries only a very small risk; but if a patient lies on a table and tries to visualize exactly where the long tube is going as it traverses his body, he is likely to get quite upset. The question is whether you can do a good experiment and obtain basic data necessary for your purposes if the patient lies on the table figuratively chewing his finger nails and literally shooting epinephrine out into his system.

One wonders how many of medicine's greatest advances might have been delayed or prevented by the rigid application of the rule of informed consent to research at large. Even physicians were in a sense intellectually and emotionally unprepared for the earliest triumphs with cardiac surgery. What, then, would have been the layman's reaction to a full exposition of the problems involved in the original Blalock-Taussig procedure? The benefits of cardiac catheterization have quite appropriately won Nobel Prizes for three of the physicians who pioneered in its use, but it is not difficult to imagine lay journalists dubbing the early experimentation barbaric and Nazi-like.

Dr. Ignacio Chávez of Mexico City has reminded us:

In the last century, it was still said that the surgeon who operated on the heart deserved the contempt and condemnation of his colleagues. This was, of course, on account of the risk. The first person who tried to do it would be an investigator conducting an experiment on a human being. The day finally came when daring surgeons tried it. . . . Can one say that they violated the norms of professional ethics when they exposed their patients to dangers which, though unknown, were unquestionably very grave? Can such an experiment . . . be considered unjustifiably daring? At the time, there were among their amazed contemporaries many people who thought so, especially as with each new step forward, the death roll grew. For one patient whose life was saved, several others died during the experiments. Was it right to go on?

... Where did one draw the line between the justifiable and the unjustifiable?

It has been argued that the fact that an unethical experiment ends happily does not exonerate the scientist who planned it. The philosophy that the end does not justify the means could be implemented in a variety of ways, including the refusal of the scientific community to recognize publicly the results of such experiments, as by denying them publication in medical periodicals. Such a view has the merit of both high principle and consistency. But if an unethical group of researchers were to stumble upon a cure for cancer of the lung, should we pretend that the data did not exist? Should we be willing—for the sake of one principle—to discard the principle of using all available knowledge to save a life? By so doing, doctors might acquire just as much guilt as the original culprits.

It has also been argued that the magnitude of risk and of potential gain is irrelevant, and that one cannot have different sets of rules for experiments of different kinds. And yet such a principle runs counter to common sense. A person may be annoyed by any invasion of his privacy, but the loss of a few minutes of his time in answering questions or pushing some buttons is not as serious a matter to him as risking loss of a limb, an eye, or his life. Similarly, it is inconceivable that serious risk can be accepted if the potential gains of an experiment are trivial.

Where does consent begin and end in a clinical trial? During the field trials of the poliomyelitis vaccine, there was some risk not only to the child given the polio injection, but to neighborhood children who might get the disease from the injected child. It might have been argued that one should require consent from the parents of the children who were not vaccinated, but it was decided not to do so.

The use of children in such trials poses serious legal and ethical problems. Some physicians allege that no such experiments are ever justified. They have found an ally in New York

State Senator Seymour Thaler, who in 1967 introduced a bill, as an amendment to the state's rights law, that would nullify written consent by a parent or guardian to permit a minor (under twenty-one) to participate in medical research except in an emergency or under court order. The result would be, in the words of one pediatrician, to make "therapeutic orphans" out of children. A child will never be able to benefit from a new drug if it cannot be tried on him. The fact that the drug works in adults will not be recognized by the FDA as valid evidence for its efficacy and safety in children. Some diseases are unique to children, or occur primarily in the pediatric age groups, and therefore cannot be studied effectively, or at all, in adults. Polio and measles vaccines might never have been developed under such restrictive measures. At the other extreme, equally benighted, is the notion that pediatric research is in no way different from other investigation, and that parental consent in such cases is no more involved than the signing of a slip granting permission for one's child to be operated upon.

If we are concerned with the problem of risk and danger, rather than the abstract trampling of human rights, we will need to invoke the principle of consent in a host of other medical situations. The use of many old drugs, as well as many surgical techniques, both old and new, involves risks greater than those obtaining from the application of many investigational drugs. If we are to rely on informed consent rather than the good judgment of the trained physician, we shall have to reorganize completely the practice of medicine.

What of the surgeon who is about to do his first heart surgery in humans? Should the patient, or the patient's family, be told that although the procedure is an accepted one, this surgeon has only performed the procedure a few times in dogs? *Someone* has to be his first patient, if he is to be added to the national pool of experienced surgeons, just as some patients have to be cared for (under supervision, to be sure) by brand-new interns every July 1.

In my own experience as a physician and investigator, not only are patients usually unqualified and unable to make the decisions, but they usually do not want to make them. A friend once called me in considerable anxiety because his physician had disclosed to him the controversy over the use of long-term anticoagulants in the management of patients who have recovered from a heart attack. The friend protested that he was in no position to judge whether his wife should receive anticoagulants, that he really would have preferred his physician to make the judgment.

The use of volunteer subjects or patients who are not actually being treated for a specific malady with the new drug under investigation must surely involve informed consent in the fullest sense possible. The volunteer subject or patient is not presented with a set of balanced alternatives. He stands to gain little or nothing from being exposed to an investigational compound, and he may run considerable risk. In such studies, the investigator has a particular responsibility to avoid the abuse of such patient groups as the mentally defective, the psychiatrically ill, and the dying. Some would deny the right of society to use prisoners as volunteers, but I have not been able to perceive a convincing argument behind such a position. This is a "captive" group in a very special sense of the word, but if handled properly there need be no more abuse of prisoners' rights than those of any other group of volunteers, who are all captive to something, even if only a sense of guilt or the need for money.[4]

In most clinical situations, by contrast, the principle of consent is much more difficult to apply and should be approached with an open and flexible mind. The investigator will have to weigh closely a number of factors, including the psychological makeup of the patient, the nature of the disease, and the possible dangers from the drug. In any case, whether

[4] Is there any more captive population than the family of a child requiring a kidney transplant? Should we therefore refuse such donors?

consent of some sort is obtained or not and whether review committees are involved or not, the ultimate safeguard for the patient will still be the training, conscience, and good judgment of the investigator, not laws or ethical codes.

Remarkably absent from public discussion of consent has been the widespread acceptance by citizens of other restraints of all sorts. It is an undisputed fact that society does disregard or constrain individual freedom in the interest of the majority. An accident-prone driver may have his license taken away from him, and a reluctant draftee may be asked to give up his life in a war he does not understand or support. A man's home may be condemned to destruction to make way for a new bridge or school, and his water may be fluoridated to prevent dental caries no matter how he may personally feel about the benefits or risks involved. Thus there is ample precedent—whether desirable or not—for society to impose involuntary sacrifices on the individual, and it is strange that so little attention has been paid to this aspect of the situation in research, even if exact parallels cannot be drawn.

At a meeting of the British Medical Research Council where the legal and ethical aspects of clinical trials were being considered, it was decided that there is no obligation on the part of an investigator to inform a patient that he is participating in a trial. If the trial is an ethical one and if the choice of treatment is really being made by the toss of the coin, the council considers it not the best part of doctoring to inform an ill patient that no one knows how to treat him and that the treatment is being determined by chance.

Finally, the concept of informed consent is borrowed from the field of medical malpractice litigation, where it is still a relatively new concept and where the decisions are confused and sometimes in conflict. In clinical investigation, the concept has never been interpreted or even applied by the courts. Risks and potential benefits of research must without question be balanced against each other, but weighing such risks and benefits is difficult and can hardly be legislated. Some legal experts have said that the day of the general operative consent is over, and that any patient has the right to compensation if he was not properly informed of the procedures and risks before consenting to them, no matter how careful the surgeon may have been. The consequences for the patient and doctor of such a philosophy are predictable—and perhaps we do not really desire them. The following letter from Dr. Sanford Kaminester of Brooklyn appeared in a medical newspaper, and is only half jest:

I am considering having printed informed-consent forms which I will then give to each patient with instructions to have it read by her husband and herself, signed in duplicate before a notary public, and returned accompanied by an attorney's affidavit to the effect that it has been read and understood.

For example:

"I, Mrs. Jane Doe, have been informed by Dr. John Roe that I require the operation known as hysterectomy. Since this operation cannot be done without anesthesia, Dr. Roe has explained to me that there are the following risks to spinal and general anesthesia: Sudden fall in blood pressure with possible kidney failure; infection in the spinal canal with fatal termination; permanent nerve damage resulting in varying degrees of paralysis; psychic shock inherent in being awake during administration of anesthesia and observing preparations for the operation; fatal cardiac arrest, pneumonia; edema of glottis with tracheotomy; infections at sites of injections; air embolism; allergic reactions to drugs.

"In addition, since many hysterectomies are associated with varying amounts of blood loss, it becomes necessary to understand the dangers attendant upon blood transfusions: mismatching of blood with fatal kidney complications; hepatitis, allergic reactions.

"Depending upon the type of pelvic pathology, there are certain risks incidental to the technical problems presented: hemorrhage; infections in the abdominal wall with possible hernia formation; injuries to the bowel with possible peritonitis or obstruction—these may be fatal or may result in the need for secondary operations, fistula formations, or hernias; injuries to the urinary tract, with possible extravasation of urine, peritonitis, or vesicovaginal or ureteral fistula; or, if a ureter is severed or ligated, a kidney may be lost.

"We next have to consider the possibilities of postoperative complications like spinal headache, distension, vomiting, pain, psychic trauma, drug addiction, allergic reactions, infections at the sites of injections, wrong medications, or incorrect dosages of medications either ordered by the physician or given by the nurse.

"If I escape all these posibilities, I am still subject to difficulties due to artificial menopause, shortness of the vagina with attendant marital problems, and bladder difficulties due to overdistension, catheterization, and infection.

"And finally, I will have to pay Dr. Roe for his services. This may constitute a severe emotional shock.

"I fully understand that, after I have read the above, consulted with another gynecologist to confirm the diagnosis and need for surgery and explain all the medical terms to me, my lawyer will meet with Dr. Roe's lawyer and between them, draw up a contract if I still have the courage to be operated upon.—[signed] Jane Doe."

I am sure that many readers will think of contingencies I have overlooked.

In the problems taken up thus far, the risk of legal action against the physician remains primarily a theoretical one. In other areas, however, the risk to him is more real, and the physician again finds himself torn between adherence to the law and the benefit of society. Charles Whitman, the student in Austin, Texas, who shot and wounded forty-three people, seventeen of them fatally, before his own death at the hands of a police officer, had consulted a psychiatrist months previously, at which time he expressed some thoughts about "going up on the Tower [of the University of Texas] with a deer rifle and...shooting people."

Many who read the psychiatrist's disclosures after the incident criticized him for not having revealed this information to authorities. Others came to his defense, pointing out the discrepancy between what many psychiatric patients threaten to do and what they actually do, and the legal restraints on physicians.

The American Medical Association Principles of Ethics state that a physician may not reveal confidences entrusted to him in the course of medical attendance, or deficiencies he may observe in the character of patients unless he is required to do so by law or unless it becomes necessary to protect the welfare of the individual or of the community. A breach of this law could result in a physician being censured by the AMA or expelled from it and from his state and county medical society as well. He would then risk suspension or loss of privileges at hospitals that make medical-society membership a prerequisite.

All states permit a patient to enter a suit for civil damages against the doctor who discloses his patient's confidence in violation of AMA ethical standards, which are considered the accepted standards of practice in the community. In addition, twenty-two states have laws stating that violation of the patient's confidence is so unprofessional that the offending doctor's license may be suspended or revoked. In thirty-seven states, there are laws stating that professional communications from a patient to a doctor are privileged, and may not be revealed without the patient's consent, even in court or for the patient's welfare. In most of these thirty-seven states there are exceptions to the law, most commonly when the patient has a communicable disease, when a will is being contested on the issue of the deceased patient's competence, when the patient has been the victim of a crime, and when there has been physical abuse of children. In every state the patient has the right to waive his privilege and authorize the doctor to testify or release information to a third party.

In Great Britain, on the other hand, the doctor is compelled in a court of law to disclose at the judge's direction any confidence or secret knowledge of this type or face imprisonment for contempt of court, since by common law only confidential disclosures to legal advisers are privileged from compulsory disclosure in court.

In situations that are covered by laws, a doctor may prefer to break the law, either by revealing information that he legally should not or by refusing to reveal information that he legally should. One such situation is when a doctor is called to see a patient who has had a criminal abortion. Another situation is when a doctor finds one member of an engaged couple afflicted with an inoperable cancer. To keep this from the intended spouse may be legal, but it is also remarkably cruel. Still another example of frustrating the law occurs when a surgeon finds a sponge or an instrument in the abdomen after a previous operation. Such a foreign body is *ipso facto* proof of malpractice, but it is customary for the second surgeon to remove the foreign body and say nothing to the patient.

One of the most distressing aspects of interaction between medicine and the law occurs when the physician is asked to testify in court. There are several factors that make the physician-scientist's life particularly difficult in this situation. The first of these is the U.S. adversary system, in which a lawyer operates on the basis of loyalty to his client, except for certain ethical and legal restraints. The opposing lawyer is bound by similar loyalties. But the physician is rarely in a position to speak with such total commitment to the cause of one or the other side. Occasionally the evidence is clear-cut, as in a paternity suit in which a hematologist or geneticist can say without any hesitation that the accused cannot possibly be father of the child in question. But these cases are rare. More often the physician can only express an opinion as to the true state of affairs. This is often made particularly difficult because he has not been in on the case at an early date and must evaluate data retrospectively, including the opinions and information derived from other physicians.

One may counter that such opinions are perfectly appropriate, and indeed this is what the doctor will be told by lawyers. It becomes sticky, however, when the physician has engaged in prolonged or intense discussion with capable lawyers. Some lawyers become so wound up in their cases that they categorize the plaintiff and defendant in black-and-white stereotypes. A physician can be swept along by this enthusiasm and case-building, ultimately finding himself on the stand stating things with certainty and assurance that are not at all that clear, and that he later regrets having uttered.

I participated in a case in Florida in which a rather strange woman, who had good cause to resent the medical profession throughout her lifetime, died slowly and painfully of a mouth cancer, leaving several million dollars to a hospital rather than to her relatives. The experts who testified on behalf of the family trying to break the will obviously visualized the deceased as a mentally unbalanced woman whose precarious mental state was further addled by the drugs she was being given to control her pain during the last months of her life. The opposing experts saw her as a reasonably well-balanced woman who could not possibly have been affected by the drugs she received. The judge, in his wisdom, threw out all the expert testimony, feeling that the experts on the two sides completely neutralized each other and that the case would have to be decided on other grounds.

The strains of testifying in court dissuade many physicians from acceding to the requests of lawyers to provide expert testimony. The medical profession is well aware of the small number of physicians within its ranks who provide biased or false testimony for a fee. These unethical doctors link up with unethical lawyers, with very little benefit to the court or the cause of justice, but a great deal of benefit to the pocketbooks of the physicians in question. In spite of such distasteful examples of the doctor-witness, however, medical testimony may be necessary or appropriate, and if all physicians avoid court testimony, where will the judges and juries of the land receive medical judgments? As may already be evident, and will perhaps become clearer during the course of the next chapter, collaboration between the legal and medical professions has not been ideal. Both professions are at fault, but society pays the price.

15

The Law
and the Patient:
Friends or Foes?

THE DIFFICULTIES in reconciling the philosophy of the law and that of science were most pungently exemplified in my own life by an incident that has been called the Great Aspirin Explosion—or, as one friend preferred, Ad astra per aspirin.

Some years ago television viewers were first told, by the manufacturers of Bayer Aspirin, of a scientific study, sponsored by the government and published in the *Journal of the American Medical Association*, purporting to show that Bayer Aspirin is unsurpassed in efficacy and safety. The scientific report was even referred to in the 1963 annual report of Sterling Drug Inc., in which can also be found the following proud statement: ". . . a notable performance by Bayer Aspirin in the United States where consumers gave our No. 1 product an impressive vote of confidence in the form of the largest dollar sales gain for any year in our history."

The story behind these events begins in the late 1950's, when the Federal Trade Commission became concerned over the frenzied increase in advertising of painkillers competing for the consumer's dollar. Once upon a time, ads for aspirin-type analgesics were moderately restrained. Bayer had a large corner of the market, and Empirin, another tremendous seller, didn't even advertise to the lay public. The advent of St. Joseph's Aspirin took over a good portion of the children's aspirin market, but the battle began in earnest after the introduction of Bufferin.

Bufferin rode to popularity on the basis of unequivocal claims that it worked faster and with less irritation to the stomach than did "unbuffered" brands of aspirin. The Bayer people, stunned, began underwriting studies of the problem. They concluded that such "buffering" was a gimmick with no clinical implications. Their scientists periodically checked the composition of Bufferin tablets, and found the percentage of ingredients changing perceptibly from time to time, without any apparent rhyme or reason. The only clear fact was that none of the recipes seemed capable of neutralizing much stomach acid. (Alka-Seltzer is the only popular aspirin preparation that does.) Lacking any clear justification for putting out a buffered aspirin, Bayer saw no reason to change its product. But Bufferin continued its hold on a large part of the market.

The frenetic advertising campaigns of Anacin and Excedrin further increased the tempo of the multimillion-dollar struggle, as blatant TV advertising brought success to these two products as well. At this point, the Federal Trade Commission started to build up its case against the widespread advertising excesses. Superficially, it would have seemed an easy thing to do. Since each drug manufacturer was implying that his brand was better and safer than any other, most of them had to be wrong. (As an FTC attorney put it: "At worst I can only lose on one of the indictments.")

But things are not always what they seem. The FTC had to prove that the advertising was deceptive, not simply demand evidence from the manuf eturers to substantiate their claims. Accordingly, the government patiently began to solicit reputable clinical investigators to check the claims made for the various products.

At this point another physician and I were asked to study the analgesic efficacy and side-action liability of several over-the-counter aspirin-type remedies. Our first reaction was less than enthusiastic. It seemed likely that we would detect no differences. The scientific value of such a study would be small. On the other hand, we suspected that many people were spending up to four times as much money as they needed to for a given amount of pain relief. We finally agreed to perform a study as a public service.

The study showed that Bayer Aspirin, Bufferin, St. Joseph's Aspirin, Anacin, and Excedrin were almost equally effective as pain relievers, and that with the exception of Excedrin and possibly of Anacin, the incidence of reports of upset stomach was not any higher after these pain relievers than after milk-sugar tablets.

In November 1960, my colleague requested permission from the FTC to present our data for scientific consideration at the annual meeting of the Committee on Drug Addiction and Narcotics of the National Academy of Sciences–National Research Council. The director of the FTC's Bureau of Investigation responded that he was "mindful of the keen interest with which the Committee is likely to receive [the] report" but had to refuse permission because premature disclosure might adversely affect any planned regulatory action. Two years later, it seemed unreasonable to delay further scientific summarization of the findings, and we again requested permission to publish. This time it was granted. The paper was submitted to the *Journal of the American Medical Association* and promptly accepted. Once again there was a quiet period, while the manuscript was being processed.

Then, around Christmas of 1962, things exploded, even before the article was printed. The AMA publicists recognized that the report had news value, and prepared advance press releases. The makers of Empirin (which we had not even studied) were upset because the article seemed to indict acetophenetidin, an ingredient of Empirin. This was because an abstract added to the paper in the editorial offices of the *JAMA* pointed out that the two preparations associated with a higher incidence of upset stomach contained acetophenetidin.

A more distressing event was the request of the Bayer folk to purchase thousands of reprints of the *JAMA* article. Someone in the company had contacted a secretary in the *JAMA* offices and asked how much it would cost to order 150,000 reprints. Having been given a cost figure, the company assumed that the reprints could be ordered, and that they could use such reprints in an advertising campaign. Fortunately, very large orders for *JAMA* reprints are automatically routed through the editor's office in Chicago for approval, and I was contacted for permission. I refused.

Next I was visited by Dr. Theodore Klumpp, the president of a subsidiary of Sterling Drug, makers of Bayer Aspirin. Dr. Klumpp enjoys the reputation of being a statesman in the pharmaceutical industry because of his long experience in the field and his former position as medical director of the Food and Drug Administration. Our chat was most amiable. Dr. Klumpp argued that the reprints would merely go out to physicians without further comment. He was delighted that a capable group of investigators had published findings exactly similar to those his company had been accumulating for years. Why not set the record straight with the doctors of America?

I explained that it was contrary to the policy of our group to allow our scientific communications to be used for commercial gain by anyone. Dr. Klumpp said that he couldn't quite see things my way but respected my decision. I thought the matter closed. To my great shock, there shortly followed a cyclonic nationwide campaign of Bayer advertising, based on our paper, including full-page ads in 188 newspapers in 98 cities, as well as radio and television spots. At the end of the newspaper ads was an invitation to write in for a free reprint of our paper.

My only consolation was that Glenbrook Laboratories, the division of Sterling Drug responsible for the ad, would be embarrassed by their inability to fill requests for reprints. I reckoned without proper appreciation for the ingenuity of today's businessman. Glenbrook proceeded to buy up *JAMA* issues and tear out our article. This must have taken a bit of doing, because one of my colleagues, writing from his home address, did not receive his "reprint" for some four months. On learning what had happened (the AMA admitted selling 2,500 copies of their total of 3,300 extra copies of the issue to Glenbrook) I complained to the manufacturers. A Glenbrook vice-president replied: "I am pleased to inform you that our supply is exhausted."

Bristol-Myers, makers of Bufferin and Excedrin, felt called upon to get into the picture after Sterling wrote a "Dear Doctor" letter to physicians calling our study to their attention. Bristol-Myers was not content to question the validity of our observations and the wisdom of generalizing from one patient population to the entire universe of people with pain. They could not refrain from pointing out that the Bayer ads had elicited a Federal Trade Commission complaint "in almost record time."

And so they had. There was hell to pay at the FTC when the story broke. One reason was that the article had tipped the hand of the commission. More important, since the FTC had approved publication, was the fact that the study and the government were now being used for profit by one of the companies whose ads had started the FTC attack on analgesic promotion.

The ads claimed that a "government-sponsored medical team had compared Bayer with four other popular pain relievers and reported in the highly authoritative Journal of the American Medical Association that the higher priced combination-of-ingredients pain relievers upset the stomach with significantly greater frequency than any of the other products tested, while Bayer Aspirin brought relief that is as fast, as strong, and as gentle to the stomach as you can get."

The government argued that the conclusions of the clinical investigators were their own personal opinions and had not been endorsed or approved by the government, by the American Medical Association, or by the medical profession, and that several of the scientific claims made in the ads were unwarranted on the basis of the reported study.

The initial request for a temporary injunction to prevent further advertising of the sort in question was denied by Judge Archie Dawson, of the New York Southern District Court, on March 8, 1963. His decision was appealed. Circuit Judges Smith, Kaufman, and Marshall of the U.S. Court of Appeals considered the case carefully and concluded that Judge Dawson had not been "clearly erroneous" in finding as he did. Their decision makes interesting reading.

The judges observed that "it is not difficult to understand the heart-warming reception this article received in the upper echelons of Sterling and its Madison Avenue colleagues . . . believing that the Judgment Day had finally arrived and seeking to counteract the many years of hard-sell by what it now believed to be the hard facts." They went on to restate the basic principle of the Federal Trade Commission Act: that the consumer has the right to rely upon representations of fact as the truth. The jurists remarked:

> . . . unlike that abiding faith which the law has in the "reasonable man," it has very little faith indeed in the intellectual acuity of the "ordinary purchaser." The general public has been defined as "that vast multitude which includes the ignorant, the unthinking and the credulous. . . . The average purchaser has been variously characterized as not "straight

thinking," subject to "impressions," uneducated, and grossly misinformed . . . influenced by prejudice and superstition; and [one who] wishfully believes in miracles . . .

They also observed that "we have come increasingly to recognize that 'advertisements as a whole may be completely misleading although every sentence separately considered is literally true.' "

After this deceptive start, the learned judges then proceeded to demolish the government case by analyzing the ad for "the average reader" (even though the FTC works on the basis that the ad must be judged in terms of its impact on the most ignorant and foolish of readers) but acting as if their own skeptical analysis was typical of what most people would think.

It might be argued that the justices were correct in assuming that no reader would interpret the ads as implying governmental or AMA endorsement of the findings (although I find it an unwarranted assumption), but one can take issue with their conclusions in terms of their own guidelines. Their opinion contrasted the present situation with that in the case of some Old Gold cigarette ads thrown out as misleading in 1950: "Although the statements made by Old Gold were at best literally true, they were used in the advertisement to convey an impression diametrically opposed to that intended by the writer of the article."

As one author of the aspirin article in question, I at least feel qualified to comment on this latter aspect. There were at least three claims or implications in the ad that rubbed me the wrong way. The first was that our study showed the pain relief from Bayer Aspirin to be as "gentle or as fast as you can get." The second was that Bayer Aspirin is as "gentle to your stomach as a sugar pill." The third was the statement that the fifteen-minute pain relief performance of Bayer Aspirin was better than that of the other products. My fellow author and I specifically stated, in a letter published in *JAMA* on March 23, 1963, that we (along with other doctors) firmly believe that any brand of aspirin can cause gastric irritation and bleeding. There are analgesics available that are certainly less irritating to the stomach than aspirin. One can also get faster and better pain relief from a shot of morphine. Finally, we had specifically stated in our article that the edge in pain relief held by Bayer at the fifteen-minute mark was slight and not significantly different from that of the other products.

On July 10, 1963, a Federal Trade Commission hearing examiner dismissed the government's complaint, concurring with the decisions of his predecessors. The matter was taken up, in writing, with the National Association of Broadcasters Code Authority and with the National Better Business Bureau at their request. Members of these bodies were sympathetic, but the results were the same: no change in the ads.

From the consumer's standpoint, the outcome of this comedy of errors was not wholly undesirable. The Bayer people unquestionably make a satisfactory brand of aspirin. They boast of more than a hundred laboratory tests to "insure the uniformity, quality, potency and purity" of their product. It is cheaper than most of the widely selling drugs competing against it, although it is more expensive than the cheapest aspirin you can buy. Thus the net impact of our article and the Bayer campaign rewarded indirectly millions of consumers who were spared some side effects from more complicated mixtures, and who saved some money they would otherwise have spent on the more expensive products sold by Bayer's competitors. From the standpoint of the scientist on the firing line, however, one might quietly have asked whether the legal decisions in this case really made sense.[1]

A PARTICULARLY difficult question is the role of the physician in the courtroom when the issue is the presence of insanity. Con-

[1] In July 1967 the Federal Trade Commission proposed new regulations aimed at ending deception in advertising claims for nonprescription analgesic drugs.

sider the fundamental question of whether a person can assume the role of defendant in a trial initiated by the state. The person is declared incompetent if he is unable to understand the proceedings against him, and decision as to the guilt or innocence of the accused cannot be made at such a time. Instead, the patient is committed to a state hospital until he is restored to "reason." This finding of incompetency is made with the aid of psychiatric testimony, which in some states is obtained by appointing physicians to this task and in others is provided by experts who amount to hired partisans testifying for a given side.

But psychiatrists are asked to conduct examinations without being given any guides about what competency to undergo a trial actually amounts to. To quote Dr. Jay Katz of Yale:

> What should we listen for when we interview a person to determine competency to stand trial? Do we evaluate his behavior in the interview situation, his diagnosis, his prognosis, his social values? If, at present, we accept such an assignment and make what is often called a routine psychiatric evaluation, do we not forget that a trial as well as the rules which govern trial practice have no analogue in clinical psychiatric practice? And can we ever make any kind of psychiatric examination without first being clear for what purposes we are conducting it?

Since normality and mental health are almost impossible to define from either a statistical or clinical viewpoint, normality depends on what the function is, and what the audience for the act is to be. For Western cultures, losing possession of one's faculties is evidence of a psychiatric illness. This is not the case in less sophisticated societies, where trance states are not exceptional or unusual phenomena but experiences witnessed, if not actually undergone, by most members of society.

Over a decade ago, in a New York trial, two psychiatrists testified that the accused was unable to stand trial and two others claimed that he could, although all agreed that the accused was a manic-depressive. The psychiatrists who thought the accused to be competent believed that although he claimed to be the Messiah, with supernatural vision and mission as well as powers, he was still able to confer with counsel and to understand the nature of the proceedings against him. The court, confused by the conflicting expert opinions, chided the experts, resentful at finding itself in the position of acting as the judge of the facts at issue as well as of the law.

Underlying this brouhaha among lawyers, judges, jurors, and psychiatrists is the very real problem of how to restrain individuals who are feared as being both crazy and criminal. The waters have been muddied in recent years by several unorthodox approaches to the problem of mental illness and the law. Dr. Thomas Szasz, a professor of psychiatry at the State University of New York in Syracuse, seems to believe, for example, that there is no such thing as mental illness, that all criminals should be considered responsible regardless of their mental state, that enforced hospitalization is rarely necessary and then only for brief periods, and that hospital psychiatry is a form of legal despotism. Dr. Szasz would eventually do away with all forced psychiatric hospitalization, would consider all wills valid regardless of the testator's intellectual competence, would allow judges to grant the death sentence to convicted murderers on request, and would allow anyone to injure himself or commit suicide if he so desired. Dr. Szasz considers psychiatrists hired henchmen who are sought by husbands and wives to "dispose of their adversaries." He has compared psychiatry to slavery. Dr. Szasz maintains that abuse of the rights of mental patients often violates the fourth, fifth, sixth, seventh, eighth, thirteenth, fourteenth, and fifteenth amendments to the United States Constitution.

There is something to be said for his position. Many patients are committed to psychiatric hospitals without having been apprised of their legal rights as to communicating with the outside world, filing writs of release, and so on. Some voluntary patients have their status changed to that of medically certified patients while in the hospital, rather than being allowed to leave the institution and to be returned as committed patients. In many jurisdictions, criminal defendants are all too quickly declared incompetent to stand trial and are then summarily committed to a psychiatric hospital without trial. Some share Dr. Szasz's concern about giving a "neutral" court psychiatrist the sole and final responsibility for important decisions, without any sort of appeal mechanism.

Unlike Dr. Szasz, with his commendable concerns, there is a lunatic-fringe element that considers the whole mental-health program of the country inspired by subversives and in fact an enormous Communist plot. One psychiatry professor wrote of receiving a letter that said, "Caesar had his arena, Hitler his gas ovens, Russia her slave labor camps, and the Kennedy Administration its mental-health institutions." Since some of our psychiatrists are foreign-born or foreign-trained, crank "200 per cent Americans" have published pamphlets saying, "In the United States today a large percentage of the psychiatrists are foreigners. MOST OF THEM EDUCATED IN RUSSIA. THE PERCENTAGE RUNS AS HIGH AS EIGHTY."

These individuals are obsessed with the notion that many patients are railroaded into hospitals as part of a sinister persecution, designed to achieve some political or religious end. In the state of Utah, the following amendment was actually offered to one of the mental-health bills: "It shall be a felony to give psychiatric treatment, nonvocational mental health counseling, case finding testing [sic], psychoanalysis, drugs, shock treatment, lobotomy, or surgery to any individual to change his concept of, belief about, or faith in God." This amendment was passed by the Utah House of Representatives and requires that no person can receive treatment under the act without the signed permission of a clergyman of his choice and of his next of kin. A pamphlet published by the Patrick

Henry League says, "The history written by the Mental Health crowd has been one of subversion of truth, disregard for human rights, and repeated association with Communist causes."

As the eminent criminal psychiatrist Manfred S. Guttmacher pointed out, many members of the legal profession do not see the serious, recidivistic criminal with a severe personality disorder as one who is emotionally deformed and socially crippled, but merely as a "bad guy." In their eyes, such an individual needs only to make the attempt to go straight.

While many lay persons, including prosecutors, will admit that the homosexual pedophile may be incapable of social restraint, they are unwilling to make the same assumption for a burglar. It seems to be a case of being incapable of identifying with the first type of offender, because most people cannot conceive of a constant urge to be sexually involved with small boys. The psychiatrist may feel that a burglar is under the sway of impulses just as powerful, abnormal, and incapable of control as the pedophile, whereas the layman considers burglary the result of laziness, a lack of desire to work, and greed.

Dr. Guttmacher eloquently made a case for the humanity of institutionalizing some individuals whose impulses are beyond their control. He cites the example of a man originally referred to a court clinic at the age of forty for murdering a young prostitute whom he had known for only a few hours and whose body he had hacked to pieces. The verdict was second-degree murder, but Dr. Guttmacher in his report to the court stated: "There is a very striking sadistic component in his personality, which he exhibits particularly toward women. This crime is the culmination of these sadistic impulses." The man was sentenced to ten years in the penitentiary, but got time off for good behavior. Thirteen years later he was convicted of assault and sentenced to eighteen months in prison, having inflicted a severe laceration of the neck on the male friend of a prostitute to whose room he had gone, possibly for the purpose of committing a crime similar to his first. Seven years later the man committed a second murder, beheading a prostitute in order to fit her snugly into an available trunk. With proper legal action, the second murder would have been prevented, provided one accepts the premise that there are people who are criminally insane.

Dr. Guttmacher was prominently involved in the trial of Jack Ruby. He pointed out that many factors were working against Ruby in Dallas. Because the death sentence was being sought, people who opposed capital punishment were eliminated from the jury. This tended to exclude jurors likely to be sympathetic to psychiatry and its methods. Guttmacher found Ruby to be a very sick man, with recurring instability and irrational outbursts of aggression. His father was a drunken sadist, and his mother spent many years in a state hospital. He was shifted about from one foster home to another, and in 1952 had a depressive psychosis. Electroencephalographic studies by a scientist from the University of Texas showed evidence of epilepsy, and these findings were corroborated by one of the foremost electroencephalographers in the country, Dr. Frederick Gibbs.

In Texas, however, the law requires that when a plea of insanity is entered, it must be shown that the defendant did not know the nature or quality of his act, or did not understand that it was wrong. Apparently the Dallas jury had no difficulties in reaching a decision to condemn Ruby to death. After many days of conflicting testimony, a verdict was handed down in two hours and nineteen minutes.

As far back as the Talmud, one finds evidence that minors, deaf-mutes, and mental defectives should not be punished for crimes "because with them only the act is of consequence, while the intention is of no consequence." St. Augustine declared that insane persons "do not know what they do, their offenses come from necessity and hence they are deprived of freedom of will." But there had to be overriding evidence of insanity for a society to exonerate a man.

It is said that in ancient Athens an ax was convicted of injuring a citizen, taken to the edge of the city, and cast away, and in Leyden, at the height of the Renaissance, a dog that had killed a man was sentenced to be hanged. (This was apparently not purely a retaliatory move, since it was decreed that the animal was "to remain hanging in the gallows to the deterring of all other dogs"!)

Our legal system has been hamstrung since the mid-nineteenth century by the so-called McNaughton[2] rule. Daniel McNaughton was a Scot who in 1843 killed Edward Drummond, the secretary of Sir Robert Peel, having mistaken him for the Home Secretary. He was found not guilty on the ground of insanity, a verdict that created a furor. The House of Lords voted to take the opinions of the judges on the law governing such cases, and the judges pronounced the following: "To establish a defense on grounds of insanity, it must clearly be proved that, at the time of committing the act, the party accused was laboring under such a defective reason, from disease of the mind, as not to know he was doing what was wrong." The British Commonwealth and most of the states have made the McNaughton rule the foundation of the laws on criminal responsibility. Many psychiatrists feel that only the grossest of psychoses can qualify a person as suffering from "McNaughton madness."

This rule was promulgated in an age when a psychology akin to phrenology was in vogue. The mind was viewed as made of discrete elements, neatly partitioned from one another, rather than an integrated unit of amazing complexity. The test of responsibility also makes use of ethical terms and concepts alien to the work of a psychiatrist in his daily examination and treatment of mentally disordered patients. The psychiatrist does not particularly seek to learn about his patient's knowl-

---

[2] The name is spelled in all sorts of ways, but the man's signature and the documents in the London Public Record Office without exception use the form "McNaughton."

edge of right and wrong, since he lacks any unusual competence to make judgments in these areas.

In 1963 the English Criminal Law Revision Committee
recommended the abolition of the verdict commonly referred
to as "guilty but insane." Two years previously, the Lord Chief
Justice had drawn attention to the fact that injustice may result
because no appeal is possible from a verdict of "guilty but
insane." The committee recommended that the defendant
should be able to appeal against a special verdict of "not guilty
by reason of insanity." The appeal could be directed either
against the finding of insanity, or against the implied finding of
the accused guilty of the act charged, or both. The committee
further recommended that when in a trial for murder the
accused pleaded either insanity or diminished responsibility,
the prosecution should be allowed to adduce evidence tending
to prove that the act had been performed. The committee also
recommended that the defendant should be able to appeal not
only from the finding that he is fit to plead, but from the finding that he is unfit to plead.

It has been suggested that psychiatrists could best assist
the courts in their deliberations by not being required to express an opinion as to the defendant's responsibility. Instead,
psychiatrists should merely state whether the defendant was
suffering from a mental disorder, how and why that conclusion
was reached, a description of the effects of the accused's disorder on his judgment, self-control, and behavior, and whether
the alleged act could be considered typically symptomatic of
the disorder.

Some have argued that it is immoral to punish unbalanced
offenders, even if they qualify as responsible under current
legal tests of responsibility, and that the law should concentrate
on dangerousness, deterrability, and treatability, and dispose of
the defendant on the basis of these criteria rather than responsibility. Still others would abandon completely the plea of in-

sanity, recommending instead that a trial merely determine whether the defendant had committed the prohibited act; the defendant would then be studied by a group of behavioral experts who would prescribe the disposition best for society and for the individual. Both Professor Katz at Yale and the chief justice of the New Jersey Court of Appeals have come out for this radical departure—which does not make clear how one acts when the best interest of the individual and of society are in conflict.

It is unreasonable to claim that no person who commits a crime should be held responsible for it. Most criminals are not sick in the sense of showing significant mental deviation from a broadly defined normal. In addition, certain kinds of crime, such as rape and income-tax evasion, are probably deterred by penal sanctions. Yet most sex offenses against small children and most murders are probably not deterred by punishment of any kind, including capital punishment. In juvenile courts, judges usually make no attempt to assess responsibility or even culpability, since the child's social maladjustment is considered largely the result of constitutional factors, parental influences, and social forces.

There has been considerable discussion in recent years about what kind of restraints society may exert on the mentally ill. This has ranged over what kinds of institutions and what length of time are appropriate, what crimes and mental illnesses deserve such restraints, and at whose initiative and at what stages of the criminal process these restraints should be invoked.

The problem is complicated by the inadequate facilities for treatment in many of our state mental hospitals. The law does not recognize that the patient has a legal right to treatment, but it has been suggested that constitutional due process of law should allow the release of an institutionalized mentally ill person if he is not receiving adequate psychiatric and medical care and treatment. Most courts and physicians reject this notion, probably for reasons similar to those of the New York Supreme Court judge who said: "Counselor, if you are really suggesting to me that I should let a crazy man out of a state hospital while he is still crazy merely because he is not getting proper care and treatment, then I think that you must think that I am crazy to even suggest this to me. Also, I am wondering if you are crazy to seriously suggest this to me."

Nevertheless, the commitment rates in different parts of the United States vary more than 800 per cent, and these variations from place to place and time to time do not seem related to variations in rates of incidence and prevalence of severe mental illness or to levels of care and treatment given to inmates in institutions. One must conclude that there are many severely mentally ill persons who in a certain community and at a certain time would not be committed, and would be allowed to remain in the community, whereas in another community or at another time they would be committed for institutional care and treatment. Does society have the right to sentence a mentally ill person to prolonged hospitalization for therapy that is not forthcoming?

WHILE IT IS NOT desirable for the law to lag behind medical knowledge, it is equally dangerous for the law to get ahead of such knowledge. One possible instance of the latter situation is the current widespread legislation on screening for phenylketonuria (PKU). This disease was first identified as a syndrome of mental retardation associated with phenylpyruvic acid in urine. At present, however, the diagnosis of PKU is based on a chemical analysis of the blood, and there are laws in the majority of our states that provide for screening programs, compulsory in most cases, based on such analysis.

It is still unclear, however, whether all individuals who

have the untreated chemical disease are or will become mentally retarded and whether the lowering of high blood phenylalanine concentrations by a diet deficient in this amino acid from birth or early infancy will necessarily prevent mental retardation in the full-blown disease.

Many people with normal intelligence have now been discovered who have blood concentrations of phenylalanine in the range found in patients with severe mental retardation. Screening programs are uncovering two to three times as many "abnormal" individuals by plasma concentration of phenylalanine as were found previously by evidence of mental retardation. The question has therefore been asked, especially by Dr. Samuel Bessman of the University of Maryland, whether these extra "phenylketonurics" will really turn out to be retarded at all. It is conceivable that there are fifty people in the population with only one defective gene for this disease for every person with two defective genes, and if some of these so-called heterozygotes handled phenylalanine poorly at birth, they would have a high blood concentration of the amino acid, and the "disease" would be diagnosed even though they were really normal mentally.

Whether an excess of phenylalanine in tissues actually causes postnatal deterioration in man is also under debate. The IQ of a child with PKU does indeed fall with the passage of time, but this is seen in almost every form of congenital mental retardation, including children with hydrocephalus and mongolism. In a sense, there is a built-in progressive drop in IQ tests in all retarded children, since the tests measure learning versus time, and retarded children fall progressively behind normals as they grow older. The seizures formerly considered to be caused by high concentrations of phenylalanine in the blood are now also recognized to be capable of remitting spontaneously, independently of the plasma concentration.

While it has been claimed that dietary treatment is beneficial to children with a high phenylalanine level, certain psychological tests show significant drops in the first year despite dietary therapy. Statistics do show an average IQ 40 points lower for institutionalized mentally retarded patients with PKU than for children who had high plasma phenylalanine concentrations at birth and were placed on special diets, but it is impossible to dissociate the effects of diet from the effects of intellectual stimulation at home, and the dietary treatment may also have placebo effects. (Children with mongolism given placebo therapy, for example, have been reported to show mental improvement greater than a control group given no therapy at all, and the potentially deleterious effects of institutionalization of mongols are generally accepted.) In view of all this, it seems reasonable at least to keep an open mind as to the benefit of restrictive diets.

Furthermore, there are worries in regard to the possible harm from deprivation diets. It is generally assumed that such diets are harmless, but there is a large body of nutrition research indicating that severe deprivation of any essential amino acid may lead to mental retardation, growth failure, and death. Several deaths have occurred during therapy of PKU with a deprivation diet, and many instances of severe reaction to phenylalanine deficit have been reported in PKU patients. It is probably extremely important to monitor plasma concentrations of this amino acid to regulate therapy, since the possibility exists that indiscriminate application of deficient diets may result in more harm than good. (The harm may also be easy to miss. If a person with a potential IQ of 110 drops to 90 because of malnutrition, who would know? He is still normal, even if less intelligent than he should be.)

Unfortunate, too, is the fact that the actual methods for measuring plasma amino acids are difficult to perform, and at least three methods in general use frequently disagree in their results.

The effect of PKU legislation has thus been to enforce upon the public a treatment program similar to the highly rational vaccination for smallpox or the administration of eyedrops to newborn infants to prevent certain kinds of infectious disease, but based on dubious evidence. It is possible, in Dr. Bessman's words, that society has been asked to "crystallize our medical ignorance into law," and that this legislation, intended to abolish PKU retardation, may on balance paradoxically act to society's detriment.

16

The Many Faces of Drug Abuse

For years I have aggravated the already difficult lives of medical students by refusing to define "drug addiction." Instead, I have emphasized that the term may represent one thing to a pharmacologist, another to a law-enforcement officer, still another to a sociologist, and quite another to the addict. The tremendous complexity of the problem of drug abuse is in fact a key issue, because it dooms to failure any simplistic, all-purpose approach. The social problems of drug abuse are so obviously multigenetic, and the manifestations so highly varied, that the solutions must be both multiple and imaginative if they are to succeed.

It is provocative to suggest that there are no addicting drugs, but only drug addicts. Like most aphorisms, this one is a good deal less profound than it sounds. But it has a point to make: that it is more important to focus on the person than the drug. Consider some of the known facts. First, a given dose of any drug will produce markedly different results in different subjects. Second, even among the members of a socio-economically deprived city ghetto group, not all individuals will try narcotics, and of those who do, a sigificant number will not continue their use. Third, and perhaps most impressive, is the phenomenon of the multiple drug user, the person who experiments with one drug after another, or with several simultaneously, in a restless search for pharmacological solace. Since these drugs vary enormously in their biological impact, it is more reasonable to find the motivation in the psyche than in the chemicals.

The history of narcotics usage began when man first learned that there were natural products available, the oriental poppy among them, to ease his pains. Over the centuries, opium[1] evolved into a household remedy, a mainstay of the physician, a medium of exchange, and a form of self-indulgence as a confection or for smoking. Until the latter half of the nineteenth century, there was little recognition of the possibility of overindulgence in its use. Instead, it was considered a panacea for most ills. Such addiction as occurred caused no social concern. No prescription was needed to obtain opium, which was freely available in grocery stores. Patent medicines for cough and diarrhea and soothing syrups for children contained opium.

American attitudes toward addiction changed because of three developments. The first was the reform movement that culminated with the passage of the first national Food and Drug Law in 1906. The manufacturers of nostrums containing opiates were portrayed as evil men, the public having been aroused to the dangers of proprietary remedies. Since the manufacturers were evil, it seemed rational to conclude that the persons who took the drugs were also bad, or at least that the habit was undesirable.

The second factor was the Civil War, which occurred shortly after the invention of the hypodermic syringe and needle. Wounded veterans became addicted as the result of the

[1] Opium is the collected and dried juice that exudes from the incised ripe poppy head.

injection of morphine for the relief of pain, and addiction was actually so common that it was termed the "soldiers' disease." Many veterans remained addicts until death, but since these men had been given drugs for the treatment of wounds suffered in the service of their country, they were usually regarded with compassion rather than scorn or contempt. The continued use of morphine by injection among these addicts, however, was possibly a cause for concern and revulsion.

The third factor was the entry into the United States of some 70,000 Chinese laborers between 1852 and 1870. Many of these were opium smokers, since this relatively benign practice was a normal part of their culture. The Gold Rush led many gamblers, criminals, and sporting types to the West, and some of these began trying opium. Opium smoking spread rapidly among antisocial, delinquent individuals, the amount of opium imported into the United States increasing from 20,000 pounds in 1860 to 298,000 pounds in 1883. Since most of the American opium smokers were criminals or near criminals, the public began, quite irrationally, to conclude that opium smoking was responsible for the antisocial behavior of these people.

More important in some ways was the change in attitude toward the Chinese. These hard-working, honest people began to induce resentment as soon as the Western railroads were finished. They opened shops, started laundries and restaurants, and became serious economic competitors, since they were willing to work for lower wages than whites were. The depression of the 1870's only made the situation worse, and race riots against the Chinese occurred in California and Canada. The "yellow peril" hysteria culminated in the Chinese Exclusion Act of 1888 and brought to the social attitudes toward opiate addiction a new tinge—that of racial prejudice. Opium dens were pictured as lurid hellpots where white youths were deliberately debased and white women enticed into prostitution. This factor of racial and national prejudice was further strengthened after 1900 by the fact that large numbers of addicts were of Italian, central European, or Jewish descent, and since 1950 by the realization that most addicts in the slums of our large cities are members of the Negro and Spanish-speaking minorities.

The rational handling of addiction has also been hampered by two lurid contributions to public attitudes: the entry of criminal types into the supply end of the producer-to-consumer chain, and the fact that some drug users have been romantic literary figures such as De Quincey, Coleridge, Baudelaire, and Cocteau, whose imaginative descriptions of their own drug experiences reflect less the pharmacology of the situation than the flamboyant personality of the writer.

The Harrison Narcotic Act was passed in 1914 in order for the United States to fulfill its obligation under the Hague Convention, which was attended by most of the nations of the world. These nations agreed to limit production and trade in opium and drugs derived therefrom to the amounts necessary for proper medical and scientific use. This law is based on federal tax power and is a system for licensing the importation, manufacture, distribution, and sale of opiates from the point of importation to the final consumer. The act provided that licensed doctors could prescribe or dispense opiates only in the course of their professional practice and to bona fide patients only, and made no provisions for the treatment of persons already addicted.

After the end of World War I, addicts were gradually cut off from their usual source of supply by the increasingly effective enforcement of the federal law. They had the choice of discontinuing the habit, seeking their drugs through the medical profession, or patronizing the illicit market. Although the last alternative became the popular solution, many of the delinquent addicts began to patronize that small minority of physicians who prescribed narcotics merely for profit. A few physicians were arrested because of these practices, and several such cases were taken to the Supreme Court, which upheld the constitutionality of the Harrison Narcotic Act.

Following World War I, there was increasing interest in narcotics legislation in the state legislatures. The Uniform Narcotics Act was drafted and adopted by the National Conference of Commissioners on Uniform State Laws in 1932, and has now been adopted in some form by almost every state in the Union. Such state legislation relies greatly on prohibitive regulations, with the ultimate sanctions being criminal penalties.

Penalties in most states are severe and have become progressively more severe in the period since the Second World War. In Illinois, selling or furnishing narcotics can call for a term of imprisonment from ten years to life for the first offense and a mandatory life term for subsequent offenses. In Pennsylvania, penalties for the same crime range from a fine up to $5,000 and imprisonment from five to twenty years for the first offense to a fine up to $30,000 and imprisonment for life for a third offense. In 1957 the Texas legislature, without one opposing vote being cast, made provision for the death penalty in certain cases of sales to minors. Many states consider convicted narcotics offenders ineligible for probation, suspended sentence, and even sometimes for parole. Federal law has so defined the criminal offense as to make it possible for an offender to violate three or more federal criminal provisions by a single illegal sale, and the Supreme Court has upheld the authority of the federal courts to impose cumulative sentences for all the offenses so committed, saying that this is consistent with the "determination of Congress to turn the screw of the criminal machinery . . . tighter and tighter."

Narcotics legislation in general deprives officials within the legal order of their ordinary powers of making decisions. The judge's ability to control his decision is severely limited in many states by the high mandatory minimum sentences and the minimal power to make use of probation. Unless he utilizes various *sub rosa* devices, the judge is likely to be hamstrung.

Police authority is abused more often in the area of narcotics offenses than in many other areas. The victim, if there is one, is a willing victim. Such a victim, or his family, is unlikely to denounce the offense or volunteer information or assistance to the police in apprehending the offender. As a result, detection of vice-squad crimes may involve violations of individual privacy, and illegal arrests, unlawful search, and improper use of undercover agents occur all too frequently.

Drug peddlers, not to be outdone by state legislatures, have on occasion resorted to their own surrealistic "legal" procedures. Attorney General Stanley Mosk of California seized a contract in a Los Angeles narcotics raid in which relations between seller and buyer are clearly spelled out in the true tradition of American business. Except for the fact that white gladiola bulbs are used to refer to heroin capsules and tulips to refer to pills, the contract reads very much like an ordinary business agreement.

For example, it is stated in this contract that "all purchases will be made with approved firms only, the approval of such to be agreed upon by each and every one of the partners a party to this venture." It is further stated that

> All sales will be made COD. No credit shall be extended by this organization. . . . Sales commissions shall be set at 25 per cent of the gross net profit up to a gross net profit of one hundred and seventy dollars a week. All profits above this amount shall be divided equally among the partners of this venture unless mutually agreed upon by all parties. . . . Weekly quotas shall be five thousand [heroin capsules]. . . . This venture shall be explored on the basis of loyalty and confidence. . . . All partners shall conduct their personal lives in a manner to enhance the reputation of this partnership, when such actions as they might undertake privately can be openly viewed by competitors in the field, and/or business associates.

A minority of people first become exposed to narcotics in legitimate medical situations. Those who begin to take such illicit drugs as heroin or marihuana or LSD can be motivated by bravado, defiance of society, and the desire to obtain "kicks." Alcohol, which is legally available, does not involve the same motivations. In all instances, there is a desire by the user to "get off the norm," to change his usual emotional, intellectual, or perceptual set. There is also often a tailoring of drug to personal need, since the drugs do differ in their pharmacological effects and the specific desires of different individuals will be best satisfied by different drugs.

Man is not the only species capable of obtaining pleasure from drugs. At the University of Michigan, monkeys have been allowed to choose between solutions of morphine and placebo. The majority of monkeys placed in this situation spontaneously chose the narcotic. Similar experiments have shown that monkeys will repeatedly (and often compulsively) press a lever to inject morphine, amphetamine, cocaine, alcohol, or barbiturates into themselves. They will take these drugs even when suffering significant physiological impairment from the medication. One can only surmise that the drugs provide an experience that is in some way prized by these caged animals. These experiments make one wonder about the analogy between this situation and the frustration, boredom, and sociological imprisonment suffered by many members of society.

Since only some people become compulsive users of drugs, there has been considerable speculation as to predisposing factors. In some work done years ago by a group at the Harvard Anesthesia Research Laboratory, we found that when healthy male volunteers, without knowing the specific nature of the drugs, were given such drugs as amphetamine, morphine, barbiturate, and heroin, the majority found the effects of amphetamine desirable, but only a minority enjoyed morphine or heroin. Those who described the opiate drugs as pleasurable had personality characteristics consistent with older psychodynamic formulations concerning the personality of the drug addict. These particular subjects were immature, dependent personalities, unrealistic in their goals, narcissistic, high in anxiety and hostility, and impatient at delays in the immediate gratification of their desires. We concluded that given equal opportunity for exposure to drugs, legal or illegal, certain individuals will treasure the effects of narcotics more than others, and will be more likely to seek such drugs illicitly.

The figures on the magnitude of our national narcotic problem are grossly inadequate and imprecise. One problem lies in what one's definition of an addict is. Does a person who occasionally uses heroin qualify as an addict? If this is the case, and one includes all the individuals who are unknown to the law officers of the country because they have never been caught, the national figure is considerably higher than the 50,000 or so that is usually cited, although it is still minute compared to the number of people who indulge in alcoholic beverages.

At present, most heroin users are in their teens, twenties, and thirties. Why are there comparatively few older users? Some die from infections caused by the circumstances under which they take narcotics or of overdose, or because they have inadvertently taken the wrong drug. Others commit suicide. Some are dropped from the narcotics rolls because they are in prison. Others probably become adept at outwitting the police. It has been suggested, nevertheless, that there is a "maturing out" of opiate addicts. According to this theory, the typical drug user begins at adolescence or in his teens, using opiates as a replacement for decisions concerning vocation, school, and starting a family. By his thirties, such a person drifts away from drug use, because the pressures of authority and law enforcement eventually have a greater impact than in earlier periods. This situation is similar to the case of juvenile delinquents and psychopaths, two groups in which the majority of individuals seem ready for more normal living by the time they reach their thirties.

In contrast to the period before World War I, there are at present substantially more men than women users, with a ratio estimated at anywhere from three to one to five to one. Urban areas show a high concentration of addicts, probably for a variety of reasons. Drug usage is connected with conditions of human misery. High addiction areas are those traditionally associated with low socio-economic status, and with environments where a highly congested minority group lives in an atmosphere in which there is ready access to illicit drug supplies and which encourages individuals to experiment with drugs.

The typical user in recent years has had no established vocation, although some occupational groups are said to be overrepresented, including jazz musicians, physicians, and nurses. In one study of 409 jazz musicians in the New York City area during the mid-1950's, 24 per cent were described as occasional and 16 per cent as regular users of heroin, with a considerably higher usage of marihuana. It is estimated that perhaps 1 per cent of the 200,000 physicians in the United States are addicted to opiates. The American Nursing Association receives annual reports from state licensing boards on nurses who have lost their licenses as a result of using opiates illegally. This number has ranged between 50 and 100 in recent years, but since nurses can probably conceal their drug use even better than physicians, it is likely that these figures are misleading.

Isidor Chein and his colleagues at New York University have performed some of the most sophisticated studies on the phenomenon of narcotics use. The high cost of heroin, the drug generally used by juveniles, forces specific delinquency against property for cash returns. Since the juvenile addict is young and unskilled, crimes like burglary and prostitution are committed in order to obtain funds.

Not all juvenile users become addicts in the usual sense of the word. In one sample of ninety-four heroin users who were members of antisocial gangs, less than half used the drug regularly, even though most of them had been on the drug for more than a year. A third showed a decrease in the frequency of use.

Escaping the pull of the delinquent subculture requires a great determination on the part of these youngsters. A boy who refuses to engage in experimentation with the use of drugs may be labeled "chicken" or "square." Although street gangs are associated in the public's mind with drug abuse, most gangs set limits to drug use by their members, since users are thought to be unreliable "on the job" and get the whole gang into trouble if arrested. The formation of little cliques to take care of the specialized activities of users threatens the cohesiveness of the gang as a whole. Almost all juvenile users get their first dose free from someone in their own age group; they are not initiated into the habit by an adult narcotics peddler.

Not all juvenile users come from the most deprived conditions. Some are from better-off families within the high-risk areas (and of course some are from well-to-do families in good neighborhoods). All the juvenile addicts, however, are in Chein's opinion severely disturbed, and the causes of personality disturbance can be traced to family experiences. The addict's family is likely to be pessimistic and distrustful, and the addiction-prone youngsters live always on the periphery of a delinquent subculture, most users having friends who have been in jail, reformatory, or on probation. These youngsters feel anxious about facing adulthood and its problems, and heroin reduces the pressure of the addict's personal difficulties. The drug habit causes the members of delinquent gangs to participate less and less in gang warfare, joint trips to movies, and sports, and more and more in gang-organized robberies and burglaries. The interest of these juvenile addicts in girls decreases, and they often give evidence of homosexuality in their behavior.

By contrast, physicians generally become addicts first in the mid-thirties, after five to ten years of busy medical practice. The doctor addict has often had an unsatisfactory relationship with his parents and childhood difficulties greater than those usually experienced. He becomes discouraged about the anticipated rewards of medical practice and disillusioned by the lack of help he has obtained from marriage and by his inability to grow into the traditional role of father and parent. Some have chronic somatic illnesses. Narcotics provide a feeling of gratification and satiation and temporary freedom from tension and frustration. Despite the high incidence of narcotics addiction in physicians, however, this group is probably the most successful in dropping the habit.

Once started on drugs, there is an important positive gain for most individuals who continue to take drugs. I have known busy lawyers and executives who used narcotics as tranquilizers to take the edge off an unbelievably high-powered and tense professional practice. Other individuals enjoy the fantasy life possible under the influence of opiates, daydreams that range from making millions of dollars to being the champion prize fighter of the world. Narcotics also insulate a person from his environment, diminishing not only anxiety but feelings of sex and hunger. In the Andes, peasants chew coca leaves under situations of extreme physical hardship, treasuring the effects of cocaine in reducing fatigue and in combating hunger on the long trips over the mountains. Truck drivers use amphetamine-like drugs primarily in order to stay awake on long trips, whereas adolescents relish the "high" obtained from such drugs. The strange assortment of people who have taken LSD for kicks ranges from severely disturbed individuals to bored young thrill seekers.

Part of the urge to continue taking certain drugs can be traced to physical dependence. This refers to certain symptoms that become manifest when a drug that has been taken steadily for a prolonged period is suddenly withdrawn. The pattern varies from drug to drug both qualitatively and quantitatively. With narcotics the withdrawal symptoms are not usually life-threatening, but they are sufficiently unpleasant to provide a strong stimulus to seek out a continuing supply of narcotics. Even here, the problem is complex. Some addicts who have access to adequate quantities of narcotics purposely withhold the taking of drugs until the withdrawal syndrome has reached a dramatic peak, and draw an analogy between this phenomenon and the eating of a beefsteak when one is ravenously hungry as opposed to when one has recently eaten.

Some fascinating experiments suggest that psychological conditioning may play an important role. Certain addicts state that even after prolonged abstinence from narcotics they feel a desire to take drugs, almost as if they were suffering physical withdrawal symptoms, if brought into contact with individuals whom they associate with the taking of narcotics in the past or with a physical environment where they have taken drugs before. This is corroborated by observations on rats addicted to narcotics. These rats show a variety of manifestations on withdrawal of narcotics, including something called the "wet-dog" syndrome, which consists of the rat shaking itself as a wet dog does. These rats not only "wet-dog" after immediate withdrawal of narcotics, but also at a later date if they are merely placed back into the environmental cage where they underwent the symptoms of withdrawal.

From time to time, newspapers report that some youngster or an important figure in show business or the sports world has been found dead under mysterious circumstances, and the diagnosis often is revealed to be acute overdosage of narcotics. This is at times traceable to a more potent supply than usual of heroin, but may also represent suicide or the injudicious administration of overdosage under conditions of alcoholic or other intoxication. In some cases, the autopsy findings suggest a shocklike syndrome due to sensitivity to the drug. Alcohol and barbiturates, singly or together, can also cause death if taken in overdose. Drugs such as LSD, cocaine, and amphetamine may induce acute psychotic episodes during which the individual harms himself or others.

Another hazard is that of withdrawal symptoms. Whereas with heroin or morphine the syndrome is usually unpleasant but not dangerous, and for cocaine and amphetamine remarkably benign, consisting essentially of a period of sleepiness and depression, those who undergo withdrawal from serious alcohol or barbiturate addiction run a 10 to 20 per cent chance of death. This withdrawal syndrome takes the form of delirium tremens, often complicated by repeated grand-mal convulsions.

A third hazard is from infections. This is most common in narcotics addicts, where it is usually related to the use of un-hygienic equipment, often shared by a number of users. Needles, syringes, and solutions of drug may become contaminated with various kinds of organisms. As a consequence, there is invasion of the bloodstream with microorganisms, with resultant sepsis, infection of the heart valves, malaria, or hepatitis. There may be phlebitis or infections of the skin, including tetanus. For the female addict, there is the added risk of venereal disease acquired via the prostitution in which she may engage in order to raise money to feed her habit. In alcoholics, infection is most often in the form of pneumonia or lung abscess resulting from aspiration of vomitus following a period of intoxication. The use of so-called blue velvet, which is a preparation of pyribenzamine dissolved in paregoric, can lead to thrombosis of the pulmonary capillaries from the talc present in the pyribenzamine tablets.

Nutritional deficiencies, cirrhosis, and a strange form of cardiac degeneration may supervene in the alcoholic, but are not a problem in most drug abusers. The patient who is addicted to alcohol or barbiturates may also suffer trauma to bones or brain during periods of acute intoxication.

Finally, the addict is, of course, liable to legal hazards for intoxication, possessing or peddling narcotics, stealing, prostitution, or physical assault.

WHILE NARCOTICS and LSD abuse have gotten the most publicity in recent years, alcoholism is our primary national drug-addiction problem. In New York and California, there are more than 8,000 alcoholics per 100,000 population. The figure for the United States as a whole is a little over half this figure. Alcoholism is the tenth leading cause of death for all ages in California, most of these deaths being associated with cirrhosis of the liver.

In the United States, three out of every eight arrests are for drunkenness. Over half of the American population consumes alcoholic beverages of some kind. Most of this is in the form of beer, but in 1960 the average annual consumption of distilled spirits and wine was a gallon per person. In San Francisco and Los Angeles, the average family spends 5 per cent of its total expenditures on alcoholic beverages. At large university and city hospitals, alcoholism is a problem in at least 10 per cent of admissions.

Unfortunately for the alcoholic, emergency-ward treatment of the intoxicated patient is difficult. The alcoholic tends to be dirty, disheveled, disturbing, and demanding. He is typically admitted during the early hours of the morning, which does not endear him to the medical and nursing staffs. Ideally such a patient should have much personal attention, but often the choice is between diverting a large percentage of the energies of the medical and nursing staffs to his care and placing him under strong restraints and sedation, which is both cruel and less than optimal in terms of his medical needs.

If the alcoholic is lucky enough to get over his acute intoxication, delirium tremens, infection, or any other illness that was responsible for hospitalization, he rarely finds himself in an effective program for prolonged medical and psychiatric care aimed at curing his basic addiction. Whereas most alcoholic clinics are directed and staffed by psychiatrists, almost all alcoholic patients seeking medical assistance for symptoms of acute intoxication or alcohol withdrawal are treated by general practitioners or internists. Thus there has been little integration of the talents and interests of medical specialists in the treatment of alcoholics. Many of those who run therapeutic programs for alcoholics have also tended to lack objectivity, and to be evangelists rather than scientists in reporting the efficacy of their programs. The medical literature is full of dozens of cures for alcoholism, none of which has stood the test of time. Even in the case of Alcoholics Anonymous, which claims to be reasonably effective, data on actual performance are hard to obtain.

The situation with barbiturates is pharmacologically very similar to that with alcohol. Sociologically, however, the situation is quite different. Since barbiturates cannot be purchased freely, there is much less experimenting with barbiturates than with alcohol. While a black market in barbiturates unquestionably exists, and cases coming to the attention of the police usually involve black-market sources, the physician is likely to see barbiturate intoxication most often as a result of the legal prescribing of drugs by physicians for the relief of anxiety and tension. These patients come to the doctor's attention because of acute intoxication or chronic deterioration in mental functioning, or because sudden withdrawal of the agents has resulted in delirium tremens, hallucinosis, or convulsions. As with alcohol, it is better to prevent this potentially lethal situation than to treat it. No patient who is on substantial amounts of barbiturates or similar sedatives and minor tranquilizers should have these drugs abruptly discontinued; instead the dosage should be gradually tapered. Abrupt withdrawal can cause permanent brain damage from protracted convulsions or even death.

Probably no drug has received more lurid treatment than marihuana. The literature on the subject is extraordinarily contradictory, perhaps because the drug is taken in different forms, by different routes, and in different strengths in various parts of the world. The best data on American consumption indicate that this drug is not habit-forming, at least in the sense that its regular use fails to produce tolerance and its abrupt cessation does not lead to a withdrawal syndrome. Despite these facts, it has been termed an intolerable evil, indiscriminately lumped with morphine and heroin as an evil drug, and similar legal punishments are invoked for all of these agents.

Marihuana is ordinarily inhaled via the smoking of "reefers." Its effects are those of exhilaration, some perceptual distortions, a loss of inhibitions, and a changed sense of time, and they are obviously pleasant to some individuals. These effects are in many ways similar to those produced by alcohol. While individuals from cultures that prefer whiskey or gin to marihuana tend to deplore the use of the latter drug, countries where marihuana is culturally approved do not agree. In 1894 the Indian Hemp Drug Commission stated that moderate use of marihuana did not produce significant mental or moral injuries, did not lead to disease, and did not lead to excess any more than did alcohol. Many years later, in New York City, similar conclusions were reached on the basis of an experimental study and from an examination of the violent crimes committed in that city over a period of years. The casual experimentation of many college students over the years also suggests a rather undramatic vice. Marihuana's effects, like those of the opiates, are mainly in the direction of decreasing interest in sex, rather than the opposite. During the investigation of this problem by a commission created by Mayor Fiorello La Guardia of New York City, a plainclothesman testified that upon visiting a luridly lit marihuana "tea pad" in Harlem, he was somewhat embarrassed to find himself the only person in the room who was inspecting the sexually provocative pictures tacked to the walls.

The main argument against marihuana at present is that its use precedes the use of heroin and therefore can be said to lead to heroin addiction. Logically, however, one should in that case also legislate against the use of tobacco, since cigarette smoking usually precedes marihuana smoking. The truth is rather that many individuals who try marihuana have access to heroin, try that as well, and prefer heroin because of its more powerful effects. The one major hazard from marihuana seems to be the rare acute psychotic disturbance[2] due either to idiosyncrasy or overdose. Under such influence, reckless driving or other irresponsible and antisocial acts may occur.

It has never been satisfactorily explained why the marihuana user cannot be dealt with by laws similar to those applied to persons who drink alcohol. It has been argued that the marihuana industry should be brought under control by legalization, taxation, licensing, and other devices like those used to control the liquor industry, and should be exploited as a source of revenue. If the greater evil of alcohol use is legal, and the even greater danger to health from smoking of ordinary cigarettes is legal, why, it has been argued, should marihuana smoking not be legalized as well? This might, of course, lead to use of marihuana that was as widespread as the use of alcohol, but the action would have the merit of consistency.

Great publicity in recent years has attended the illegal use of LSD. This drug might be called a modern-day Tale of Hofmann. A Swiss chemist by this name accidentally absorbed a small amount of the drug several decades ago in his laboratory, whereupon there ensued a typical LSD experience, with disturbances of thought and sensory perception. Since that time, extraordinarily little has been added to our knowledge about the drug, although the psychological disturbances described in that earliest experience have been reproduced on many occasions in many people, and a great deal of extravagant writing has occurred over the wonders of the experience and the alleged psychotherapeutic marvels that may result from its use.

The mystic experiences described under LSD are nothing

---

[2] Recently, reports of disturbed behavior after marihuana seem to be increasing, and some have suggested a re-examination of the assumption that such smoking is as benign as it has been thought to be.

new. They are in quality remarkably like those experienced by users of peyote and mescaline. What is different about LSD (besides its newness) is the fact that such very small amounts of the drug (o.1 milligram, for example) can produce effects. In many parts of the country, illicit supplies are available ranging in price from one dollar to as much as ten dollars per dose. The material is sold in the form of sugar cubes containing the drug, in gelatin capsules, and dissolved in liquid. The drug is usually swallowed, and its use in social situations is frequent. It is quite common for friends to share psychedelic drugs with each other, and frequently they are dispensed at parties much as alcoholic drinks might be.

Some individuals who use LSD-type drugs are people who are narcotic-drug addicts by preference but have tried hallucinogenic agents on one or more occasions for kicks or curiosity. These people are unlikely to use the drug with great frequency or excess.

A second group of LSD users has been described as "the professional potheads"—people who have had extensive experience with many drugs, including marihuana, amphetamine, and barbiturates, but who on the whole tend to avoid the opiate drugs. They are often arty types, beatniks, freethinkers, nonconformists, and social rebels. These professional potheads enjoy the euphoria produced by smoking marihuana and also relish and seek out the inspiration, insight, and sensory distortions that they believe the hallucinogens to produce. They seem to be constantly trying to arouse themselves from their own apathy, to make life in some way purposeful, to overcome social inhibitions, and to facilitate meaningful conversations and interpersonal relationships. These people use hallucinogenic agents mainly on weekends (which, however, often last for four days) or on special occasions such as parties. The latter might be described as "unstructured": everything from basketweaving and lampshade-making to overt sexual activities may go on. (Some individuals claim that the sexual act is height-ened and prolonged under the influence of the drug. Others find that LSD tends to suppress sexual drive and prevent climax.)

Finally, there are a few people who take hallucinogenic agents repeatedly over a sustained period of time. These people do not usually take the drugs in a group for social purposes but use them mainly as a means of obtaining some personal goal. The goal may be to "find God," achieve a "Christlike state of mind," see "reality," etc.

While these drugs might be considered habit-forming for those who relish their effects, they are not addicting in the sense of producing physical dependence. Experimentally, in both animals and man, tolerance can develop to the effects of LSD, but many users of the drug claim that tolerance does not occur in their experience and that actually one may become more sensitive to the drug with repeated use. It is perhaps possible to reconcile these observations if one remembers that most LSD is probably taken infrequently enough to preclude the development of tolerance. Another possibility is that for some the mystique of the drug-taking experience eventually becomes as powerful as the drug itself.

The physical hazards from usual doses of the drug per se are usually minimal. Changes in blood pressure and pulse occur, but are usually slight. Some persons may be so confused while under its effects and so unable to function that they experience or cause accidents; several deaths have resulted in this way. Extremely worrisome have been the reports from a number of cities on the production of prolonged psychotic reactions and persistently abnormal brain wave patterns. It is not uncommon for previously rational persons to become suspicious and withdrawn under the influence of LSD, but one wonders whether these prolonged major disturbances are not related to the fact that more and more individuals who are mentally unbalanced are being pushed over the edge of sanity by the drug experience. The risks appear greatest in subjects with excessive emotional instability and psychopathic features —just those individuals most likely to be attracted to the drug by press accounts and other publicity. The latest worry stems from the chromosomal abnormalities observed in animals and humans given LSD.[3]

Several states have now established controls over LSD to prohibit manufacture, sale, and possession of the drug except by qualified persons or institutions. Whether this will do anything more than drive the drug underground is not clear, but past experiences with other drugs suggest that the problem cannot be easily solved in this way.

It is hard to say if LSD actually has a beneficial effect on alcoholics and others with mental problems, since it has often been administered by investigators who are evangelical about its prospects. At the same time, it would seem both appropriate and important to support scientific clinical research on LSD if sensible experimental protocols can be devised in this area. That LSD has any real mind-broadening effect in the sense of providing creative insights and productivity seems questionable in view of the experiences to date, despite the fervent exhortations of psychedelic messiahs who profess to find God in their navels and eternal truth in hallucinations.

The disturbed nature of many individuals seeking pharmacological escape is evident in the sniffing of airplane glue, nail-polish remover, lighter fluid, and other organic solvents by children and adolescents. Deliberate inhalation of the solvent vapors of model-building cements and other related compounds has become mildly popular in these age groups during recent years, and has been called the juvenile's counterpart of adult alcoholism and drug addiction. Sniffers have even been known to inhale the fumes of automobile combustion by placing their mouths over exhaust pipes, if other sources were unavailable.

[3] One scientific report has described a congenitally defective child whose deformities were attributed to LSD-provoked chromosomal changes in mother and father.

The psychological results of sniffing resemble a combination of the effects of alcohol, amphetamine, and LSD. Although serious organic change does not occur frequently from such practices, there is reason to worry about the effects of these chemicals on the liver, the kidneys, the blood, and the central nervous system. In at least eight instances of death from sniffing, the child apparently suffocated while inhaling glue from a plastic bag, but in two other cases, death seems to have resulted from the glue itself.

Although the children involved (usually boys) have come from many walks of life, including so-called good families, most have had a long history of delinquency and difficulties in school and in interpersonal relationships. Nearly all have had trouble in expressing aggressive or sexual drives, and many have come from broken homes that lacked a dominant male figure in the home with whom they could identify. Glue sniffers, confused by the drug or released from their inhibitions, frequently demonstrate antisocial behavior and may commit acts dangerous to other individuals or themselves. Rape, automobile accidents, property destruction, and deliberate shootings have been reported.

The doctor, in this complicated field, must know the general background of the problem. He should realize that narcotics, barbiturates, amphetamine, and other drugs are highly useful agents when properly and legitimately used, and he must not restrict their legitimate use because of the remote possibility that an occasional person may become addicted. Many patients have suffered needlessly for hours because a nurse or doctor feared that adequate dosage of narcotics would addict the patient. The doctor must be on his guard against addicts mimicking painful or other diseases so as to obtain drugs. He must not miss the diagnosis of chronic intoxication with barbiturates and related drugs, since the patient may die if the drugs are suddenly stopped. He must resist the temptation to attribute everything that is wrong with an alcoholic or drug addict to the intoxicant, lest he miss serious infections, brain injury, or other illness.

He must face the difficulties of rehabilitating both the alcoholic and the drug addict and must seek such help as is available. The hospitalization-imprisonment at Public Health Services hospitals has not worked especially well. During their stay there, addicts are indeed given psychiatric attention, job training, and other help, but the environment is not one that is conducive to rehabilitation, and the contact with hardened pyschopaths and backsliders is hardly healthy for the younger addicts. There has been little attempt to change the environment of these individuals when they return to society. With diseases that are generated by social and personal pressures, returning an addict to the same environment from which he came is likely to result only in a recurrence of addiction.

There is a growing belief that narcotics addiction should be treated as a disease rather than a crime. Dr. Vincent Dole and Dr. Marie Nyswander have created considerable excitement in New York City and elsewhere by their suggestion that addicts should be maintained on narcotics, rather than withdrawn. In brief, their program involves the daily administration to heroin addicts, on an outpatient basis, of the narcotic analgesic methadone, building up, in most instances, to a moderately high maintenance dosage, where the addicts are then stabilized. On such daily oral methadone, it is claimed that addicts do not respond with euphoria to even large doses of heroin and thus feel no urge to seek out illegal sources of it. Further, it is said that a high percentage of those accepted into the program become productive citizens, able to find and keep jobs or to function adequately in school.

The ambulatory outpatient clinic approach to maintenance therapy of addicts is not a new concept; it was tried in the United States almost half a century ago. These earlier attempts are usually described as failures, although such pilot studies were never given a fair trial.

The notion that addiction to methadone is qualitatively different from addiction to other narcotic analgesics is not readily supported by available pharmacological and sociological data. Dr. Dole has described the typical heroin addict as a person who swings violently between withdrawal symptoms and euphoria, almost never being normal or functional. Yet the investigations by Isidor Chein and others have clearly shown a spectrum of narcotics usage in big cities as broad as the spectrum of alcohol usage. Some individuals take only an occasional fix, others stabilize at some dosage level not dissimilar to the methadone blockade program, while still others use narcotics in increasing quantities and may indeed show the picture Dole considers typical. Doctors have occasion to see patients who as lawyers, doctors, or businessmen have taken narcotics for years in a stabilized fashion, some of them functioning with great skill and competence.

"Narcotic blockade" is really another term for pharmacologic tolerance. The fact that a person on large doses of methadone can tolerate an intravenous dose of 160 milligrams of heroin without serious untoward results is no more surprising than the fact that an addict who has been on large daily doses of other potent analgesics can do the same thing. Similarly, the inability of methadone addicts to respond with euphoria or respiratory depression to heroin is neither unique nor absolute. Given a large enough dose of a powerful narcotic, a methadone addict will experience narcotic symptoms and may indeed be seriously poisoned if the dose is large enough.

On the other hand, methadone does have several distinct advantages as a narcotic candidate for maintenance therapy of the type advocated by Drs. Dole and Nyswander. It is more efficiently absorbed orally, and has a longer duration of action, than most other narcotics, and its slow excretion rate makes less crucial the omission of a daily dose, since on complete cessation of methadone, withdrawal symptoms will not begin for several days, and even then they will be mild compared to those seen after morphine or heroin withdrawal.

One must admire the willingness of Drs. Dole and Nyswander to adopt an experimental approach to the problem of drug addiction. If the addict has only two alternatives—buying narcotics illicitly or receiving them daily in a clinic—the latter is preferable on almost any count, since it would not require contact with criminals or the necessity to steal or spend large quantities of money to pay for one's habit.

In addition to diminishing the opportunities for the addict to run afoul of the law, attendance at a clinic of the Dole-Nyswander type provides the opportunity for psychiatric and other help that might ultimately make it possible for the addict to function without narcotics. At the very least, the clinic and its personnel constitute a lifeline linking the addict to society, and the results thus far suggest a considerable degree of success in the social rehabilitation of addicts voluntarily engaged in the Dole-Nyswander program.

It is unfortunate that society seems incapable of discussing narcotics calmly and dispassionately. Dr. Dole and his colleagues deserve better than to be accused of naïveté and woolly-headedness. At the same time, there have been hyperbolic claims for the new treatment by those who are fiercely enthusiastic about the approach and see in it a solution to the problems of all narcotics addicts. The truth probably lies between these extremes. Dole and Nyswander have reminded us that at least some individuals who prize the effects of narcotics can be stabilized on some dose of a narcotic and behave more or less normally and productively under such circumstances. They rightly compare this situation to maintenance treatment of a diabetic with insulin or a patient suffering from pernicious anemia with vitamin B_{12}. Perhaps it is an even closer analogy to compare narcotic blockade with the need of some schizophrenics to continue taking tranquilizers in order to prevent relapse and deterioration.

The inability of programs of this type to meet the needs of all addicts was well described in a letter from a Los Angeles doctor who told of the numerous inquiries he received about methadone blockade after an article on the Dole-Nyswander program appeared in the *Los Angeles Times*:

> When told that they would be supplied with a drug called methadone at a cost of nine cents a tablet which was supposed to replace heroin, they all asked, "But will it get me off stuff, will it dry me out?" Thirteen patients remembered they had taken methadone in [U.S. Public Health Service] hospitals at Fort Worth or Lexington, said, "Thanks anyway," and hung up. Two patients said, "Doc, at that price I'll buy all you can get me," but when told that I would supply a maximum of 15 tablets a day, and would have to report my supplying them according to California law to the Bureau of Narcotic Enforcement, they hung up. Twenty-four made appointments, three showed up. One, upon entering the inner office, grabbed a prescription pad and ran out the side door. One patient I refused to handle because he refused hospitalization and insisted on outpatient withdrawal. In conjunction with heroin he admitted to using an estimated 60 grains of pentobarbital and 500 mg. of dextro-amphetamine daily. The other patient claimed he was broke and could not even pay for the bus ride to the county hospital; in fact, he admitted stealing the car he drove to the office. He wanted a month's supply of methadone because he lived far from the office and could not make weekly visits.

Since many addicts will neither desire nor seek out ambulatory clinic treatment of this sort, society will need other approaches to the multifaceted problem of narcotics addiction. Meanwhile, we must look as objectively as we can at the problems as well as the achievements of methadone blockade, and indeed other experimental approaches.

Some doctors are trying cyclazocine, a narcotic antagonist, to prevent abuse of narcotics. Cyclazocine, if taken regularly by the addict, will diminish or prevent the effects of usual doses of the narcotic, blocking both physical dependence and death from overdose. The results thus far are only suggestive, but the cyclazocine method may work well for some addicts and has the advantage of not substituting one addiction for another.

It is not clear how much leeway the physician has in treating addicts as sick people and not as criminals. The first of the "doctor" cases tried by the Supreme Court, in 1919, dealt with a case of flagrant abuse. Dr. Webb had sold prescriptions by the thousands, indiscriminately, to any applicant for fifty cents apiece. Thus the Court was dealing with a mere peddler and not a physician taking care of the ill. The second case, in 1920, also arose out of an outrageous set of facts—a doctor who had written prescriptions for morphine by the gram, at one dollar per gram. The next case, the *United States v. Behrman*, was decided in 1922, and again the abuse was flagrant. Dr. Behrman had given a known addict prescriptions for 150 grains of heroin, 360 grams of morphine, and 210 grams of cocaine. The indictment was drawn up so as to omit any accusation of bad faith. It charged in effect that this treatment was for the purpose of curing an addict and thus its validity depended on a holding that prescribing drugs for the addict was a crime, regardless of the physician's intent in the matter. A majority of the justices, moved by the flagrant facts, ruled the indictment was good.

Following this, the Narcotics Division launched a reign of terror, bullying and threatening doctors and sending some to prison. Any prescribing for an addict was likely to mean trouble with Treasury agents. The addict-patient vanished, to be replaced by the addict-criminal.

A few years later, however, Dr. Charles O. Linder, after a lifetime of honorable practice in Spokane, Washington, was induced by one of the division's stool-pigeon addicts to write a prescription for four small tablets of cocaine and morphine. Several agents descended on his office, conducted a search, and dragged him off to jail. He was indicted, convicted, and sentenced and lost on his appeal to the Circuit Court of Appeals. He carried his fight to the Supreme Court, where he was completely vindicated. The opinion this time was unanimous and is still the controlling interpretation of the Harrison Act. As the opinion stated:

> The enactment under consideration levies a tax . . . upon every person who imports, manufactures, produces, compounds, sells, deals in, dispenses or gives away opium or coca leaves or derivatives therefrom, and may regulate medical practice in the States only so far as reasonably appropriate for or merely incidental to its enforcement. *It says nothing of "addicts" and does not undertake to prescribe methods for their medical treatment.* They are diseased and proper subjects for such treatment, and we cannot possibly conclude that a physician acted improperly or unwisely or for other than medical purposes solely because he has dispensed to one of them, in the ordinary course and in good faith, four small tablets of morphine or cocaine for relief of conditions incident to addiction. . . . This opinion cannot be accepted as authority for holding that a physician who acts *bona fide* and according to fair medical standards, may never give an addict moderate amounts of drugs for self-administration in order to relieve conditions incident to addiction. *Enforcement of the tax demands no such drastic rule, and if the Act had such scope it would certainly encounter great constitutional difficulties.*

Nevertheless, the present pamphlet of the Narcotics Bureau advising doctors of their rights in dealing with addicts ignores what the Supreme Court said in the Linder case and still paraphrases the discredited language of the Webb case.

There is a need also for investigation of the methods of such organizations as Narcotics Anonymous, Synanon, Daytop Lodge, and other groups whose records are not generally available for scientific scrutiny, but which are attempting to rehabilitate the addict in meaningful ways. In a field where so little good has been accomplished in the past, it seems inappropriate to rule out the wisdom and efficiency of any particular approach.

In dealing with drug abuse, society should concern itself first of all with the causes of addiction, not contenting itself with the secondary manifestations, and should decide what the goals are in this area. The field badly needs more data and less hysteria. We must, for example, consider the possibility that drug addiction may be an alternative to other, less desirable activity. Denying access to drugs may be beneficial for some and harmful for others. Some individuals perform better on alcohol, tranquilizers, or narcotics than off these drugs, and a stimulant like amphetamine can prevent fatigue. The latter fact does not mean that truck drivers should be encouraged to drive for unreasonable and excessive distances, but it suggests that if our society forces long overnight trips on some of its workingmen, it may be better for truck drivers to be on stimulants than off them. (Why is it heinous to take a "pep pill" but fine to swill a gallon of coffee?)

We should dissociate illegal from legal use of drugs. The outlawing of heroin from medical practice is a step aimed at controlling the illegal use of the drug, and as such is both irrational and illogical. There have never been large numbers of addicts created by the legitimate medical use of heroin, and it is foolish to act as if the opposite were true. At the same time, there are clearly criminal aspects to drug addiction, and the problems will not be solved simply by entrusting all addicts to the good offices of medical men. Many addicts engaged in illegal means of support, such as forgery, pimping, confidence games, and drug sales, reject the usual societal norms in favor of the "smart hustle" or the "cool operation." In this subculture, honest work is despised, drug use praised, and law and authority defiantly flaunted. Since there are gangsters and psychopaths involved in the illicit drug traffic, the problems call for cooperation between the law and medicine, not hostility.

Society must also stop treating certain kinds of drug abuse as atrocities. The past should have taught us that public condemnation of such ailments as syphilis and tuberculosis detracted from our ability to pick up early cases and to treat and rehabilitate afflicted individuals. If society insists on ranking evils, it would logically pay a great deal more attention to alcoholism, automobile accidents, and cigarette smoking than it does to heroin addiction.

We should try to avoid being hypocrites about addiction. Commissioner Anslinger once admitted, for example, that it was arranged for an influential Congressman who was addicted to obtain supplies from an obscure druggist on the outskirts of Washington. If this is all right for a Congressman, why is it wrong for others less privileged? Strenuously honest attempts to try outpatient maintenance therapy aimed at exactly the same goals that Commissioner Anslinger had for the Congressman addict should not be opposed. Nor do we make much progress by exaggerating the horrors of these drugs or by painting distorted pictures of the effect of narcotics use on crime rates.

Society should re-examine its legal approach to drug abuse. The current regulations at the federal and state levels are too rigid and inflexible. Many justices are opposed to the mandatory sentences and the extreme penalties now possible. The American Civil Liberties Union has suggested that the government enact provisions for the voluntary civil commitment of addicts and refrain from enacting provisions for involuntary commitment, as well as easing regulations that unnecessarily restrict doctors in administering drugs to addicts. The ACLU has pointed out that compulsory incarceration—that is, involuntary civil commitment—amounts to criminal punishment, and that commitment laws like those enacted in California and New York, providing for long periods of involuntary confinement, deprive the addict of his liberty without due process. These statutes enable the government to commit a man for cure when there has been no conviction.[4]

As Kolb has lamented: "Our approach so far has produced tragedy, disease and crime." We ought to be able to do better. At the very least, we might conjure up some compassion for the addict and drug user. In "Minutes of the Last Meeting," Gene Fowler quoted the eccentric German-Japanese Sadakichi Hartmann as follows:

> "When a man is in his dying seventies and spilling blood from every pore, struggling like a hooked shark and utterly tired of the scheme of things; what, I ask you, in the name of all the devils in hell, difference does it make if he sniffs cocaine, chews opium, smokes hashish, or has enough morphine needles to make him look like a porcupine? What difference does it make? Who cares whether you become an addict or not? Does my lack of suffering, by means of a well-placed needle, cause the government or the state any pain? Does it cause the preachers in their pulpits to swoon with severe fistulas? Does it do any harm to the Daughters of the American Revolution? . . . These may be my dying words, as indeed I hope they are; and I can assign to all the fires of hell the polliwog brains that are at the head of the so-called Health Service! Damn them all!"

In a characteristic non sequitur, he added, "If you think vaudeville is dead, look at modern art."

[4] In 1967 State Supreme Court Justice Samuel A. Spiegel declared the New York procedure for involuntary commitment of narcotics addicts unconstitutional.

EPILOGUE

O N A STIFLING day in May of 1967, several physicians (including the author) testified on behalf of Captain Howard B. Levy at his court-martial in Columbia, South Carolina. The basic constitutional question was whether Dr. Levy had the right to refuse an order violating his ethical principles.

The testimony brought out the considerable differences between Army doctors and nonmedical officers. Even in the armed forces, physicians are not just like other citizens. Traditionally, both for pragmatic reasons and for matters of principle, medicine has wisely tried to divorce itself from partisan military or political objectives. To the Army doctor, a wounded enemy soldier is a patient, not a foe; medical expertise is a bounty to be shared, not a weapon.

The Nuremberg Trials emphasized that there is a point of no return beyond which people cannot go without betraying themselves or humanity. They also reminded the world that the moral decision must be made by the individual; the state, the armed forces, or other forms of authority may command behavior that is odious, and must not be obeyed. Levy lost, as was expected, but his disobedience reminded me of the last words of a leader of the German opposition to Hitler: "The power to say 'No' in a given situation . . . is the starting point for the interpretation of man as a rational being."[1]

In a sense, this entire book is based on the premise that the physician is not like other men, that his obligations are unique and commensurate with the great power he wields over the health and happiness of his patients. It is because of his special position in society that he must concern himself not only with adequate medical care for the individuals in his practice, but with the larger public need for medical care of high quality. The threats to man from his environment, the race against famine, and the restriction of population growth are as germane to the doctor as the relative merits of oral contraceptives and intrauterine devices, the right of a woman to abortion, the right of a mongol to decent treatment at the hands of the more normal members of society. The terrors of aging and of dying, the specter and promise of heredity control, the legal rights of the sick and the mad, the needs of the drug addict and the alcoholic—all these, and much more, fall within the purview of the Compleat Physician, and for this reason have been discussed in the preceding chapters.

The philosopher Arthur D. Lovejoy once listed the requirements to be met by a scholar wishing to do an adequate analysis of *Paradise Lost*. These included expertise in English, French, Italian, classical, and rabbinical literature, medievalism, philosophy, theology, and the history of science, with special emphasis on early modern astronomy. Even a cursory look at the health problems discussed in this book should indicate the parallel demands on the doctor who wishes adequately to serve society. Ideally, he would be a superbeing rich in humanism, compassion, wisdom, logic, critique, technical expertise, scholarship, morality, honesty, political acumen, originality, legal knowledge, journalistic and oratorical skill, equanimity, a sense of history, and extraordinary mental and physical endurance.

[1] Quoted by the philosopher-historian Ludwig Edelstein.

For physicians like me—on most days I feel more like Mr. Wopsle's great-aunt in *Great Expectations*, "a ridiculous old woman of limited means and unlimited infirmity"—the task appears overwhelming. But, in the words of Albert Camus, " . . . it is not necessary to succeed in order to persevere . . . the early Christians called the great movement that sustained them 'the folly of the Cross.' "

We must, therefore, try. Our welfare as individuals and as a society is dependent on the degree to which we in the medical profession can succeed in shouldering the heavy burdens placed upon us by the environment and by our own fatuous errors, self-indulgence, and intellectual myopia.

In 1937 John Dewey addressed a group of St. Louis physicians. He told them, in part:

> We cannot understand the conditions that produce unity in the human being and conditions that generate disruptions of this unity until the study of the relations of human beings to one another is as alert, as unremitting and as systematic as the study of strictly physiological and anatomical processes and structures has been in the past. The plea is not for any remission on the side of the latter. But we need to recover from the impression, now widespread, that the essential problem is solved when chemical, immunological, physiological and anatomical knowledge is sufficiently obtained. We cannot understand and employ this knowledge until it is placed integrally in the context of what human beings do to one another in the vast variety of their contacts and associations.
>
> The one way out of the division . . . is continued and persistent study of the concrete effect of social situations upon individual human beings, and the effect, in return, of human beings upon social relations . . . in this study the physician has a position of unique opportunity and responsibility.

This book was written in the belief that Dewey's words are even more important today than they were three decades ago. It is time we heeded his message.

INDEX

About the Author

LOUIS LASAGNA was born in New York City in 1923 and was graduated from Rutgers in 1943. He received his M.D. from the College of Physicians and Surgeons, Columbia University, in 1947. He has studied, taught, and been licensed to practice medicine in New York, Boston, and Baltimore. Since 1954 he has been with the Johns Hopkins University School of Medicine, where he is an associate professor of medicine and associate professor of pharmacology and experimental therapeutics. He is a consultant to the National Institutes of Health. Dr. Lasagna is the author of *The Doctors' Dilemmas* (1962), has contributed a great number of papers to medical journals, and has written for *The New York Times Magazine*, *The New Republic*, *Catholic Digest*, and other general publications. He is married and lives with his wife and seven children in Baltimore.

A Note on the Type

The text of this book was set on the Linotype in ELECTRA, designed by W. A. DWIGGINS. The Electra face is a simple and readable type suitable for printing books by present-day processes. It is not based on any historical model, and hence does not echo any particular time or fashion. It is without eccentricities to catch the eye and interfere with reading—in general, its aim is to perform the function of a good book printing type: to be read, and not seen.

The book was composed, printed, and bound by The Book Press Incorporated, Brattleboro, Vermont.

Typography and binding design by Anita Karl.